CHICKEN THERAPY

HOW VISION THERAPY CHANGED MY LIFE AFTER A TRAUMATIC BRAIN INJURY

By Christine Louise Helm

Copyright ©2024 by Christine Louise Helm

All rights reserved. No part of this book may be reproduced, stored in a retrieval system, or transmitted in any form or by any means without the prior written permission of the publishers, except by a reviewer who may quote brief passages in a review to be printed by a newspaper, magazine, or journal.

To protect the privacy of some individuals associated with this story, their names have been changed.

It is not the intention of this book to provide medical advice. Please consult your physician with any questions concerning health concerns, including traumatic brain injury, concussion symptoms, or vision therapy.

This book is dedicated to everyone who struggles daily to find hope after a life-changing event.

ACKNOWLEDGMENTS

I would like to thank my husband for his devoted support; my daughters for being my rock; Christa Roser for her valuable input while writing this book and her dedication to promoting vision therapy; my vision therapist, Jane, for her selfless efforts to improve her patients' lives; my concussion therapist, Anita, for her support and advice; and my editor, Paul Dinas, for believing that my words could make a difference.

I would also like to thank my flock—Ike, Queen Elizabeth, Concussion Chicken, Kevin, Ruby, Lady Gaga, and Orloff—for their inspiration.

FOREWORD

When Chris told me she was going to write a book about her experience with vision therapy and how it helped her recover from her injury, I was thrilled. Not only was she planning to spread the news about the benefits of vision therapy, but she was also targeting the population of patients who often have undiagnosed vision deficits following a brain injury. After reading her book, I also realized the great impact it could have in providing inspiration to this population of patients, as well as the value of her story for healthcare professionals.

I am continually astounded by the lack of guidance in addressing vision deficits in those with brain injuries, especially considering that 60 to 70 percent of this population experience visual symptoms. Chris was one of the lucky ones who found help in Behavioral Optometry, and I praise her for her efforts in getting the word out to others who are struggling to find the help they need.

Not only will people learn about the help vision therapy can provide by reading her book, but they will also be inspired by her courage and perseverance. Chris chronicles how her vision deficits disrupted her life, including her work, her relationships, and even her self-worth. Yet she found the strength and faith to try yet another avenue of help in vision therapy, supported by her family and feathered friends.

What I was not expecting to discover in her book was the intimate insight into the struggles she was living through in her everyday life because of her vision difficulties. This book will not only be valuable in informing other healthcare professionals about the benefits of vision therapy, but also to those of us providing vision therapy for our patients who have suffered brain injuries. I have been listening to the stories of my patients for over 30 years and thought I understood what they were going through. Chris's story gave me even greater insight into the plight of the everyday for my patients.

I hope this book reaches these three populations: patients suffering from vision deficits who may be helped with vision therapy, other healthcare professionals who may be unaware of how vision therapy can help, and providers of vision therapy who may gain greater empathy and compassion from the intimate details of what it is like to live with vision deficits.

Thank you, Chris, for sharing your story.

Christa Roser, 0.0., FOVDR

Vision Therapy Associates

INTRODUCTION

Our two-story brick farmhouse, built in 1880, sits on a hidden acre on the side of a hill on the outskirts of the small Pennsylvania town I grew up in. It proudly faces south and is accompanied on the right by our yard, which is the size of a football field. The yard is dotted with trees and confined on one side by sloping woodland and on the other by our long driveway.

In late March, our woodland view comes alive with hundreds of wild yellow daffodils. In the yard, small clusters of tulips announce the arrival of spring from the edges of the flowerbeds and fruit trees.

Glimpses of deer sneaking into the yard for fresh grass, and raccoons and skunks looting the bird feeders bring my world alive. It is here where I always found comfort and peace.

Happily married, with two beautiful college-aged daughters, a successful teaching career, and a coop full of chickens and ducks, my life was complete. Our farmhouse was always occupied by family and friends. My flock of chickens and ducks freely roamed our yard, providing us with hours of entertainment and lots of eggs. Our vegetable gardens thrived.

Then, one winter evening, it all came to an abrupt halt.

A serious car accident left me with traumatic brain injuries, which included a concussion, constant headaches, muscle knots around my eyes, dizziness, nausea, and chronic double vision.

My injuries robbed me of my ability to drive, read, or work on the computer for sustained periods. I lost my teaching job. My independence and self-esteem suffered greatly. My symptoms depleted me of energy and ambition. The limited depth perception and peripheral vision made it almost impossible to navigate in any new surroundings.

CHICKEN THERAPY

Once filled with good health and rewarding activities, my life became filled with seemingly never-ending doctor visits and uphill battles with insurance companies and creditors. Seeking relief, I met with optometrists, ophthalmologists, neuro-ophthalmologists, and neuropsychologists. I was told my double vision might resolve with time but, in all likelihood, could be permanent. I was prescribed special glasses and some prescription medications.

Nothing helped.

I rarely attended gatherings with friends and stopped hosting large family holiday events. I became angry and depressed and lashed out at the very people who were trying to support me.

I filled my long, lonely days with walks around our property. The wildlife and my flock became my primary source of comfort and a welcome diversion from my depressed existence. I watched how they lived, how they died, how they reproduced, and how they survived.

At some point, I started journaling as a way of venting my frustrations. I began by writing down my experiences with my concussion symptoms. I wrote about how I felt and, sometimes, about my flock and the insights they gave me about survival. They always made me laugh and smile with their antics.

Then, with the help of a concussion therapist, I discovered vision therapy. I had little to no knowledge of this alternative therapy. None of my many doctors had told me about it.

I started to do some research on my own and discovered the power of this noninvasive, drug-free, therapeutic practice. I decided to try it. After a year, vision therapy gave me back so much of my old life by showing me how to cope with my vision issues and help them heal. It was a minor miracle.

I struggled with emotional highs and lows and blindly navigated the web of medical, legal, and insurance establishments. I began to think that my story of living with this condition could help others with similar issues by informing them about the transformative power of vision therapy.

It has taken me years to compile all my journals into this book. The process has been one of the most monumental and rewarding endeavors I have known. It is my hope that it gives you a better understanding of what life can be like for the victim of a brain injury after an accident. It is my hope that my story will help spread the word about the healing power of vision therapy.

Christine Helm

We are all searching for that answer,

The one that's in plain sight,

It's buried deep inside you,

And called your inner light.

CHAPTER 1

I grew up in the '70s. While the world around me seemed to rebel against everything, my world remained simple. I liked to follow the rules and found comfort in conformity. That said, I think I was always a sort of overachiever. If I had a slight ability to do something and a reason to achieve it, I did it to the best of my ability.

My parents married at the age of 19, as did many of their friends in 1954. A few years later, they had my sister Suzanne, and four years after that, I made my entrance. My dad had a steady job in research and development at a flooring plant, while my mother stayed at home with us. My sister and I had an ideal childhood.

I grew up in a quaint little Pennsylvania town nestled along the Susquehanna River. It was within driving distance of metropolitan cities and Amish farmland. We lived in a row home, on a block that had many families with children our ages. We walked to school and played outside until dusk. We got our allowance every Friday and attended church every Sunday. We read books and played in the rain.

School always came easy to me. Other things did not. I loved swimming and joined our local summer swim team at age eight. Although I worked very hard at practice, I never won a race. I desperately wanted to be that kid who won trophies and big horse ribbons.

There always seemed to be this spark inside me, driving me to do better. For some reason, I couldn't figure out how to harness it to swim faster. Finally, one summer day, I did.

It was a perfect Saturday morning in June of 1976. Brightly colored flags spanned the width of the near Olympic-sized pool and waved in the sunlight as it danced on the crystal-clear water below. As I stood on the wobbly wooden starting block, I knew

CHICKEN THERAPY

I was ready. All eighty-five pounds of my thin, muscular twelve-year-old body knew it too.

The sounds of timers testing their watches, parents happily chatting with one another, and the crackling voice on the PA system filled the air. "Swimmers, take your mark!" commanded the starter in an authoritative, booming voice. I drew in a deep breath to relax my nerves. I grabbed the starting block and planted my toes firmly over the edge as every muscle in my body came alive, twitching with anticipation.

The instant my ears heard the crack of the gun, my body shot like an arrow through the air, piercing the water below. Beams of sunlight magically streamed all around me as I glided through the water. Executing powerful strokes, I effortlessly flew across the pool. I had never felt more alive, so confident. By noontime, I had won three races and unofficially broken a pool record at time trials for our local summer swim team.

My ideal life was interrupted at the age of fifteen by my parents' divorce. After that, everything kept changing, and my life seemed so much harder than it was before. I slowly lost the ability to ignite my spark. The feeling I had that summer day remained elusive, while the idea of it smoldered in the pit of my stomach.

I learned to work just hard enough to get by well, managed to graduate in the top twenty percent of my high school class, and went on to a small college not too far from home. I was always strong in math and interested in tech, so I majored in computer science, a field that had been growing in importance. After my first semester, I realized it wasn't for me. Coding got boring and repetitious.

I loved to write — always had. I kept a journal during high school and worked on the school paper. Why not journalism as a major? I thought. Initially, I thrived in my classes. But after I attended a talk by a local journalist in one of my classes, I had second thoughts.

Her talk included the fact that only ten percent of writers earn enough to live on. My goal was to graduate college and earn enough money to independently support myself, no matter what. The following day, I marched to the academic advisor's office and announced I wanted to change my major.

"Well, what do you want to change it to?" mumbled the stodgy professor through the cigar in his mouth as he looked through my files.

"Something like… maybe a…" I replied, realizing I had not thought this through.

With a sigh of boredom, he continued, "Well, what are you good at?"

"Math."

"What are you passionate about?"

"Coaching. This past summer, I helped coach our local swim team to a championship. I enjoyed doing that."

"Sounds like teaching might work. You could be a high school math teacher."

I had never considered teaching. It seemed perfect. A few minutes later, I left the office smiling with a new schedule in my hand.

College graduation seemed to arrive in the blink of an eye. I anxiously awaited an interview call from any one of the ten teaching positions I had applied for. After a few interviews, I was hired to start as a math teacher and assistant coach of the swim team in another small town located forty-five minutes away. That meant I could still live at home with my mother while I ventured out into the adult world.

I never really thought of teaching as a job. It was more of a calling. After only a few years, I had become a respected, well-liked high school math teacher and coach.

Each year, I was presented with a new set of fresh minds. I quickly figured out that to succeed at teaching, I needed to continually adjust my teaching strategies to fit the needs of the class. When individual students were faced with learning or personal issues, I offered support and empathy. The challenge of successfully helping my students kept me motivated and fulfilled.

Growing up bold, beautiful, and unafraid,

Found a person to marry and a job to be enslaved,

We were all making our mark

All of our friends did the same,

Then marriage and children, and society sings…

CHAPTER 2

One Friday afternoon, I decided to accept the invitation to a friend's housewarming party. I had just completed my second year of teaching and wanted to celebrate. After the party, on the ride home, I found myself sitting beside Jon in the back seat of a friend's car.

I knew who he was but had never paid much attention. Jon did his best to act macho and tough as we conversed on the drive home. Before that night, I had never really looked at him. Tonight, I did. Jon was muscular and tall; with jet-black hair and blue eyes you could drown in.

Realizing that I had to fight to maintain the space between us because every inch of my body felt as though it was being magnetically pulled closer to him, I announced that I was tired and would like to be dropped off at home. As I was getting out of the car, Jon nonchalantly yelled out the window, "I will pick you up at six tomorrow night for our date." He hadn't asked me; he had told me. What a jerk, I thought.

"We'll see," I confidently retorted, trying to appear indifferent.

I'm not sure what I fell in love with first: his good looks or his confidence. Either way, on that first date, I fell hard and never looked back. The following year, we got married, moved into a small apartment close to home, and bought a boat. Jon worked full-time as a maintenance mechanic and part-time as a construction worker.

I still taught high school math and coached swimming in the evenings and on weekends. A year later, we had saved enough money for a down payment on a house. We bought a small half-acre property on a back road a few miles outside my hometown. Summers were spent boating with friends on the river and the bay. We were enjoying life as independent newlyweds.

CHICKEN THERAPY

Two years later, Adrianna was born. I discovered a love I never knew existed the moment she was placed in my arms. I took maternity leave and enjoyed my time with her. She had striking features like Jon and a pleasant temperament. We proudly took her out with us all the time — to dinner or shopping. People would always comment on her beauty and good behavior. Her thick, dark brown hair complemented her green eyes and fair complexion. Jon and I were sure that, together, we had created the perfect child.

When Adrianna was three months old, I found a close and trusted friend to care for her and returned to teaching. Three years and eleven months after Adrianna was born, Jade came into the world. Her beautiful little face was framed with blond hair like mine. She also inherited my brown eyes, was lively, boisterous, and a bit of a handful. We spent that year at home a lot. Jon and I soon learned that maybe parenting two small children was more challenging than we had anticipated. We also learned that spending time at home with our two young daughters made us happier than we had ever been.

Once the girls were born, life seemed to move at a much faster pace. As much as I loved teaching, I yearned to stay home with the girls more. The full year of maternity leave I had taken with Jade turned into a five-year hiatus from teaching. I tutored during the evenings and weekends and coached swimming in the summers with the girls in tow.

I clearly remember the day I noticed my handsome husband making his way to Adrianna's practice field late one afternoon in early October. The air was cool and crisp, and the warmth of the fall sun still felt like remnants of summer.

One-year-old Jade, happy, energetic, and cute as a button, was wriggling to escape my clutches as I watched five-year-old Adrianna happily gallop out onto the soccer field. Her mane of brown hair had escaped its ponytail holder and was fluttering behind her. I thought, *She is perfect.* In fact, my life is perfect. Everything I had dreamed of seemed to be falling into place.

Our little family soon became a unit. I first felt our synergy during a family vacation at a cute little bayside cabin in the woods. I couldn't wait to get away for a few days with my favorite people in the world. We had planned a week full of boating, hiking, and relaxing — just the four of us.

As we pulled up to the cabin, it appeared dirty and dingy, not quite like the pictures in the brochure. Upon entering, the smell of damp wood and something dead wafted around me. The light revealed a rustic cabin that, although cozy, appeared to have not been cleaned in quite a while. Cobwebs hung from the windows.

"Now this is real camping! Time to clean," I announced cheerily.

I was determined to make this work. Both girls happily pitched in while Jon unloaded the truck.

The next morning, we excitedly prepared the kids for their first ride on our recently purchased used boat. I wanted the girls to experience where Jon and I had spent so many wondrous summers.

The old familiar feeling of wind on my face, sun on my skin, and peacefulness in my heart was just returning when I heard the motor sputter and Jon yell. The dependable boat we were sold turned out to be not so dependable. Two hours later, we were back on shore. A boater had come upon us and graciously offered to tow us. The kids were not impressed. We headed into town with the motor in the back of the truck. Jon found a shop that would fix it. Unfortunately, it would take a few days.

Still determined to show our children how to have fun and adventure, we decided to take a hike through the woods to a well-known lighthouse. The light breeze quickly gave way to the hot afternoon August sun and biting insects. Jon attempted to save the day by inventing Indian names for all of us.

CHICKEN THERAPY

Adrianna was given the name Princess Toadpee. She had decided the night before to collect all of the toads she found on the path to the campground bathhouse. Her squeals of delight turned to horror when one of the toads she had gently lifted decided to pee on her.

Three-year-old Jade was deemed Squaw Pic Um Nose, and I was bequeathed Queen How's My Hair. Jon became King Butterfly. We made a dignified royal Indian procession toward the lighthouse, which should have been in sight by now. Only it wasn't. We realized we were lost.

After an hour, we finally found the truck, excitedly jumped in, and cranked up the air conditioning. I noticed specks of dirt on my legs and flicked them off as we went through a drive-through, only to see them reappear a few minutes later. Upon helping Jade pull up her little shorts in the bathroom, I noticed the same brown specks on her legs — a lot of them. They were not dirt; they were tiny bugs!

Back in the truck, I relayed my discovery to Jon. After a moment of silence, the rest of us peeked underneath our clothes and realized, with horror, that they were also on us. A ranger at the campground informed us that we had chiggers and that they could easily be killed with lice shampoo.

We took over the bathhouse and proceeded to smother every inch of our bodies with the shampoo we had found at a local pharmacy. The girls and I were on one side of the bathhouse, and Jon was on the other. We played Simon Says and talked through the open eaves of the bathhouse. Although this was not the day we had planned, it remains the day when we first turned hardship into happiness together.

I returned to teaching when Jade entered kindergarten. After applying to a few local high schools, I obtained a position as a high school math teacher at a nearby private Catholic high school. One of the perks of the position was that Jade and Adrianna would eventually get to attend the school for free.

It did not take long for me to adjust to the new school. I quickly became well-respected by the administration and parents. The long hours and compassion I showed my students did not go unnoticed.

It was always the problem students that gravitated toward me. I was kind and fair but did not negotiate with teenagers. I gave them respect and demanded it in return. Those who tested me quickly found themselves assigned to after-school detention in my classroom.

During afternoon detention, I would quickly address the issue and make sure the student understood my expectations. I would then passively chat with the student while correcting papers. This is when my favorite part of teaching would occur — they would eventually open up about their home life, fears, and dreams. I would learn as much from them as they learned from me.

Three years later, we decided we were financially stable enough to start searching for our dream home — a quaint little farmhouse in the country. Even though we lived in a pleasant neighborhood, we both longed to have a small property away from everything. The girls were now eight and twelve and needed more space.

One day, Jon saw what appeared to be the perfect listing and called Don, his childhood friend who was now a realtor. It was an old farmhouse in fair shape on one acre of land within our price range. We all knew the area, as it was close to where Jon had grown up and located in the girls' current school district.

That evening, Don picked us up after dark and drove us to the house. The back road leading to the house had no streetlights and was very dark. As we pulled down the fifty-yard-long driveway, the car headlights revealed a perfect two-story brick farmhouse tucked neatly beside a hill. It was surrounded by grass and trees encompassed by woods.

As we got out of the car, I gazed at the six-paned wooden windows on the front of the old bank barn embedded in the hill. Jade and Adrianna raced down the long driveway that led to a set of brick steps and down to the house. *Was it possible we could have a house and a barn? I excitedly thought.*

While we toured the inside of the house, which was in a fair amount of disrepair, my imagination gave me a glimpse of what this place could be. I could picture family dinners in the dining room and a large deck on the back of the house that would overlook the woodland below. Jon was a real craftsman, and we both had plenty of energy. I excitedly signed the paper.

In the following weeks, our entire family helped us clean up the house. My mom had the girls' rooms painted and carpeted as a housewarming gift. Although there was still a whole lot to do, the house was in good enough shape for us to move in. It was a busy but happy time for us.

So, turn off all the noise,

Sit back and unplug,

Your inner light will find that answer,

When you feed it hope and love.

CHAPTER 3

Living in a farmhouse with some extra room, we had a wonderful garden and a big yard for our dog, Riley, to run around freely. Almost as soon as we had gotten settled, Adrianna begged me to get chickens. She loved the outdoors, nature, and animals.

"Mom, we live on a farm now. We need chicks. They're so cute, and I researched them at the library. Once they grow up, we'll get free eggs."

"Maybe someday," I said. Given our busy lives, I wasn't sure we'd have the time or energy to care for a flock of chickens.

Then, a few years later, on the way back from one of Adrianna's soccer games, we passed the farm store. There was a big, hand-drawn sign on the side of the road: CHICKS FOR SALE!

"Chicks!" Adrianna said. "Please, can we get some?"

"Let's go in to look. No promises."

Jon and I had secretly been discussing the possibility of getting chickens. We hadn't told the girls, as we weren't sure we could fit anything else into our busy schedules.

Upon entering the store, off to the side, there were a few boxes filled with peeping chicks in a variety of colors.

"Mom, they're so cute," Adrianna said, kneeling to stroke one on its soft down.

I had to admit, they were pretty lovable.

Just then, a clerk walked over. "Morning," she said, smiling. "Cute, aren't they?"

"So cute," Adrianna said as she played with them.

"They're all just hatched and healthy. And they're on sale."

Adrianna looked at me, and I caved. We picked six chicks and put them in a box. We bought some food and a little booklet about how to care for them.

Once home, Jade was overjoyed. Jon shook his head and chuckled. "I guess they'll be needing a coop."

"You've got about six weeks, according to the book. Until then, they can stay in a large box with a heat lamp in the girls' room," I said.

"My room!" Jade yelled.

"No, it was my idea — my room," Adrianna insisted.

"Well, whoever keeps them needs to change the box daily," I reminded them.

"Adrianna's room!"

The girls named the chicks, and we all helped care for them. It was a happy summer. Jon built a sturdy and adorable red coop in the front yard about thirty yards from the house. The coop itself was only four feet by six feet, just big enough to house six chickens. It had two roosting bars and three nesting boxes. Chickens like privacy and small spaces when laying eggs. A small door in the coop opened to an outside run enclosed with chicken wire.

Our chicks grew to become healthy, adult hens, and prospered. We opened the door to the coop each morning so they could enjoy the outside in the safety of their run. When we were home during the evening and on weekends, we let them out of the run to free range in the yard.

Riley did a good job of guarding the property against predators. Each evening at dusk, the hens would return to the coop on their own, seeking shelter for the night. We would lock it up before going to bed.

While checking the coop late one night after a long day at school followed by Jade's track practice, we found the first egg. "It's blue!" she shrieked. We both immediately searched the internet to find out why it wasn't white and if it was edible. We learned that some breeds lay different colored eggs, but the eggs are all the same inside and safe to eat.

We also learned that all hens lay eggs with or without a rooster.

"Maybe we should get a rooster for our hens?" Jade said.

"They seem pretty happy without one," I said. "Yeah, but if we got one, we could hatch chicks, right?" We both said at the same time and then burst into laughter. "Let's do it!"

"I need to call Adrianna and tell her the news. A rooster!" Jade exclaimed as she ran up to her room. Adrianna had just started college in Pittsburgh, four hours away, and Jade missed sharing her experiences with her.

A few weeks later, we found a local farmer who was selling a young Rhode Island Red rooster. Jade and I went to pick him up. The farmer told us we only needed one rooster for our small flock of hens. He was larger than my hens, had spurs on the back of his legs, and looked headstrong.

"Well, go ahead, pick him up!" the farmer said. "He's a rooster, so you will need to let him know you're the boss."

It took all my courage, as I was slightly afraid, but I cornered him and picked him up. I was surprised at how docile and soft he was as I firmly wrapped one arm around his body and wings and the other under his feet, keeping a close eye on his spurs. The farmer helped me put him in a box with a few slits in the top.

"He will be calm in the dark box for your ride home. Separate him for a few hours, then let him in with the hens."

On the trip back, Jade named him Ike.

When we got home, we put Ike into the chicken run and let the hens observe him through the fence from afar. After a few hours, we decided it was safe to let the hens back into the run.

Almost immediately, Ike started chasing and jumping on the hens. It was chaos. The hens were racing around the run, flapping their wings and running into each other as Ike seemed to systematically jump on each hen's back for a few seconds and hold onto their comb or neck.

CHICKEN THERAPY

"Mom, he's hurting them!"

I quickly entered the run and became part of the chaos while trying to contain Ike. I realized the hens seemed not only uninjured but also unfazed by Ike's actions.

After successfully catching the excited rooster, I held him for a few minutes as he quickly calmed down, and then set him free. I explained to Jade that I had read that a new rooster in a flock would mate with each hen to introduce himself.

"You mean all that is just them mating?"

I nodded. "When males and females get together…"

"Mom…" she said, rolling her eyes, trying to sound grown up. "I know all about that."

So much for the talk.

We separated Ike again for the night with a makeshift divider Jon had built in the coop to ensure his peaceful integration and decided to let them all free-range together in the morning. To our surprise, the hens happily greeted Ike and showed him around the property. They led him up the hill, around the house, and then to their favorite dirt pile. While pecking at the dirt, Ike made an unusual sound that caused all the hens to hurriedly join him.

We watched in awe as he stepped back and allowed the hens to eat the insects he had just discovered. He was taking care of them. A feeling of contentment and understanding filled my heart. They were now a family.

Our flock grew after we adopted Ike. We initially thought our favorite hen was sick when she listlessly refused to get out of a nesting box. Queen Elizabeth was a beautiful Speckled Sussex covered in brown feathers sprinkled with white spots. She always carried herself regally and was picked on by no one.

Upon researching her symptoms, we learned that she was "broody" — a hen's natural instinct to sit on, incubate, and hatch eggs. It was the first time we experienced this. We moved her and the eggs to a dog crate on the porch to give her some privacy from the other curious hens. She remained in a catatonic-like state, which is typical for broody hens, throughout the move.

We watched with wonder as Queen Elizabeth expertly shuffled and turned the eggs every so often during the incubation period. She would shriek, peck, and puff up her feathers if any person or chicken dared to get near her. Twenty-one days later, we heard a peeping sound and saw a small head poke out from between the feathers of Queen Elizabeth's wing. By the next day, a total of seven fluffy, adorable chicks had joined our flock.

Jon, with Jade and Adrianna's help, built a small enclosure just for them that could eventually be used to house broody hens in the future. I was prepared for the extra work of caring for the chicks and was pleasantly surprised when there was none. Queen Elizabeth showed them how to eat from the feeder and drink from the waterer. I was amazed at how her maternal instincts took over. In our modern age, we are taught to rely on books, the internet, or experts for advice on everything — especially parenting and childcare. Maybe it was time for us to get back to basics and rely on our natural instincts.

When the chicks were a week old, we opened the door of their special little coop and allowed them the opportunity to explore the yard. The rest of the flock, led by Ike, excitedly ran to see the new chicks. They screeched to a halt when Queen Elizabeth puffed her feathers and made a loud shriek. Her large, angry appearance clearly communicated that they could only watch from a distance.

Like all mothers, she was protecting her children. I could relate, remembering how protective I was — and still am — of both my girls. I would stop at nothing to protect them. No one had taught me that.

The next day, we noticed that Ike, now aware of the new additions to the flock, would trot to the chick enclosure to observe them as soon as the big coop was opened in the morning. I was in awe of his attentiveness, like any proud dad.

Soon, we were up to fifteen adult hens. Not long after, proud of our experience with chickens, we thought it would be a good idea to add ducks to the flock.

We purchased five ducklings, without knowing their breed or sex, at the local feed store after doing minimal research on how to raise ducklings. *After all, we thought, how different could it be from raising chicks?* As we learned, it was a whole new ball game.

Ducklings grow much faster than chicks and create a smelly mess with the water bowls needed for them to dunk their heads. We moved them into a bathtub for their daily swims, which were necessary for their health.

Six long and exhausting weeks later, the ducklings had grown into ducks and were ready to move to the coop. Jon installed baby pools for them to swim around in. Much to our surprise, the chickens showed little interest in them. Even Ike took them in stride.

After they were fully grown, we figured out their breeds and sex. Sally, Jack, and Sandy, our favorites, grew up to be tall and skinny Indian Runners. Brie and Gouda were Muscovies. They got their names after they tried to steal my cheese and crackers one afternoon.

Whenever they were let out of the run, they stuck together, wandering the entire property and even venturing into the woods, quacking amongst each other the entire time. Unlike the chickens, they hated returning to the coop at night and had to be corralled.

Each night before sundown, we would search for and find our gypsy band of ducks and slowly herd them toward the coop. The Indian Runners would defiantly quack for the entire walk and rarely tried to get away. The Muscovies would join the group with comical hisses and tail wags.

After a few months, the females started to brood, and soon there were almost two dozen new ducklings to care for. Jon had to expand the coop to accommodate them. Watching Sally and Sandy proudly lead the twenty-one ducklings around the yard was delightful. They strutted with their heads held high past the hens, past the rooster, through the gardens, across the deck, and toward the baby pool.

The ducklings obediently followed, nervously looking around and peeping. Our entire family would stop for a moment to reverently observe this marvelous parade.

We are all waiting for that something,

Quietly in the wings,

That one thing that will make us,

The big break that will complete our dreams.

CHAPTER 4

While I always appeared confident on the outside, on the inside, I constantly wondered if I was a good enough wife, mother, and teacher. I was 50 years old, happily married, with two beautiful daughters, friends, family, and a successful teaching career. Yet, I couldn't shake the feeling that I needed to be more.

One day, while house cleaning, I came upon an old brown file folder that was secured with a ribbon. As I unwound the ribbon and reached inside, the feel and smell of the paper took me back to my high school days when I would sit in my bedroom long into the night and write in a journal. I would pen my fears, dreams, and deepest secrets. I would contemplate the meaning of life and surmise my conclusions. I would then carefully tuck those thoughts away in the brown folder, meant for only me.

As I rifled through the yellow-lined pages, now thin and delicate with age, I found a poem I had written. The poem described a person who was not afraid to step out of their comfort zone and go after their dreams — me. I was surprised by how elegant the words looked on the paper and how they flowed when I read them. *Had I achieved my dreams? What happened to that spark I embraced as a twelve-year-old?*

When the principal approached me with the idea of becoming the school's technology integrator, in charge of the school's one-to-one digital program, I jumped at the chance.

The one-to-one program would begin the following school year. Each student would receive an iPad. My role was to create the policies associated with student ownership of the iPads and successfully deploy them. I also oversaw the training of the staff on the new educational technologies.

I was always good with technology and had often helped my colleagues and students with educational software and personal devices in the past. This position opened a new set of responsibilities and included a handsome pay raise. Although I would still teach two or three math classes, most of my day would be spent developing and implementing the new program. I knew the hours would be longer, with nearly half the time spent working on computer screens, but Adrianna was in college and Jade was in high school, so I had more free time.

After accepting this offer with Jon's encouragement, I immediately took every educational technology class available locally. I applied for and was accepted into a master's program for technology education, where I would attend classes one evening a week starting the following school year. It would take a few years to complete the program, but the schedule was doable.

Freshman orientation sessions occurred during the two weeks prior to the first day of school. During the orientation, I handed every new freshman an iPad. I then taught the parents and students the setup procedures and guidelines for using their iPads.

Early on in my teaching career, I had learned to carefully prepare and be knowledgeable about any topic I presented. I confidently gave instructions and then walked around the room helping students with their problems. The evening classes, though sometimes chaotic, were always successful.

Once school was in session for the year, my days started early and ended late. Each morning, before leaving for school, I would open the door between the coop and the run and take a few minutes to watch our large flock of nearly three dozen chickens and ducks push, shove, and flap their way into the outside world of their enclosed run. I'd feed and water them, then head off.

The upperclassmen regained possession of their old iPads during the first week of school. My days started early and ended late as frantic students wandered into my room with password problems, software problems, boyfriend problems, and even uniform problems. I thrived in the fast-paced, unpredictable environment.

Many days, I would eat lunch in my classroom to accommodate the stream of students who used this time to seek my help. I tried to eat in the faculty room at least twice a week. My lunch period was scheduled at the same time as a few of the more upbeat teachers, and we enjoyed each other's company. My little group of friends at the lunch table would eagerly listen to my stories about my life or the antics of our little flock. Sometimes, they laughed hysterically.

The first two years of my new position went by in a blur. Jon and I had settled into a new routine and were enjoying being empty nesters. By my third year as a technology integrator, I had the system down, a lot of classes under my belt, and a new confidence that made my days less stressful.

Adrianna had graduated from college with honors and immediately obtained a prestigious job in Pittsburgh, four hours away. Upon high school graduation, Jade also decided to go to school in Pittsburgh. Unhappy with her course of studies, she decided to put school on hold, move in with Adrianna, and help manage a Chipotle. Even though I missed them, I was happy that my girls were experiencing independence with each other.

Jon had gotten a new job fixing and maintaining ozone-generating machines all over the East Coast. The salary was great. The downside was that he was on the road several days a week. We had never been apart on a weekly basis for so long, and it took time to adjust. On the days he was gone, it was a challenge keeping up with chores and caring for our huge flock before and after my ten-hour workdays.

It took a few minutes every morning, an hour in the evening, and extra time on the weekends to take care of the flock. We never intended to have this many birds. The chickens were one thing — they needed to be let out of their coop into the run or the yard each morning. In the evening, eggs were gathered, and waters were checked. Coop cleaning and trips to the farm store for supplies were done on the weekends. Jon would do maintenance on the coop and run once a month.

Initially, the addition of a few ducks added only a little more work, as they needed a baby pool to keep their feathers healthy and clean. Chickens took dust baths in the dirt to stay healthy. Now, several dozen ducks needing daily access to multiple freshwater baby pools presented even more maintenance.

With Jon away so much, and the girls on their own, we sadly decided that it was time to sell the twenty-one now-grown ducklings and keep the rest. I found a lovely older couple to buy them — they had a lake and a special house for ducks.

The evening before the dreaded early morning pick-up was rainy, and the run was muddy. I needed to get the ducklings into dog crates, and I had just finished a long and tiring day. Chickens are simple to catch once they settle down on their roosts. They become slightly catatonic and can easily be picked up and handled.

Ducks, on the other hand, sleep anywhere they damn well choose — with one eye open. You cannot sneak up on a duck. Catching a duck requires wits, reflexes, and defiance. I was normally up to the challenge, but this evening, it made me sad.

The evening after they were gone, I struggled to ignore the loss I felt as I fed the now smaller flock. It reminded me of the emptiness I felt when Adrianna and Jade moved out.

Afterward, I took a stroll around our property. Daisy, the feral cat who had recently adopted us, accompanied me. Throughout the years, various animals seemed to show up on our little farm at just the right time. We meandered a few yards into the woods. I watched her as she played, hiding and then pouncing at something, grateful for her company. I stayed outside a little longer than usual, hoping to find a bit of solace.

CHICKEN THERAPY

Dusk was my favorite part of the day. There was a calm at this time of day. The soothing sounds of birds settling down for the night and chirping insects slowly dissipated as the sun bowed its head. Everything was peaceful for just a moment when day and night would exchange places. Dusk was the morning of the night.

One night, when Jon was away, after eating dinner by myself on the deck, I headed to the coop to close it for the evening. Unable to shake the empty feeling I had, I tried to concentrate on the task at hand. The sun had not yet set, and the flock was foraging around outside the coop, preparing to retire for the night.

The ducks tended not to wander as far now that the ducklings were gone. Queen Elizabeth didn't like their evening presence and kept chasing them away from her peaceful hunt for bugs. Ike joined her — he seemed to like the Queen best of all the hens.

Once the chickens and ducks had retreated to the coop for the night, I did my usual head count. Four young hens were missing. Searching the property, I found them perched on a low branch in the big oak tree.

"I guess they decided to change things up!" I chuckled.

As I shooed them back to the coop, I thought: *Maybe I should change things up when Jon is away.* I decided to create a new routine of my own on the evenings he was traveling — taking it a bit easier, not trying to do it all. Although I still missed him, I began to enjoy my evenings alone and my new routines.

From this dark and lonely wing,

I view the show called life,

Patiently quelling feelings of jealousy and hate,

For those who got it right.

CHAPTER 5

It was the end of the first week back to school after Christmas break. I was more than ready to go home when the bell rang at 3 p.m.

As I packed up to leave, an odd feeling overwhelmed me. It made me stop and pause. I turned around and, with a sweeping glance at my classroom, etched the memory of this moment into my brain. I remember wanting to take it all in — the sights, the sounds, the smells, and the feelings. Having no clue why I felt this way at that moment, I immediately turned my thoughts to the task at hand: meeting Jade to pick Jon up at the airport.

It was a cold, dark, rainy January evening — the kind that chilled you to the bone. On the way to the car, I quickly shooed Sally and Sandy from a mud puddle, herded them into the coop with the rest of the flock, and locked it tight.

I smiled as I hopped into the passenger seat of our new SUV. My beautiful, sassy, now 19-year-old Jade offered to drive. She had moved back home last month to regroup after a lot of changes this past year. I admired her ability to pick herself up and change directions and was thrilled to have at least one of my girls home again.

Her laughter and love of life always lit up a room, and tonight it filled the car. Jon had been away for a week, and I was anxiously awaiting his return. After twenty-seven years of marriage, the spark was still there.

We were running late. Jon had sounded tired and stressed on the phone when he called before he boarded his flight. He had been to yet another training session for his new job on the other side of the country this past week. The classes were grueling, and the material was technical. Jon was a hands-on person who did not thrive in a classroom environment.

CHICKEN THERAPY

"Please drive a little faster," I said. "We're going to be late. It's okay if you drive a few miles over the speed limit."

Jade rolled her eyes. "I'm a safe driver. I'd rather be careful. It's the first time I'm driving this new car."

I sighed. "Okay. I just know your dad wants to get home, and I don't want him to have to wait too long."

We happily went over the details of our plan to hold up the sign we had made earlier that evening — JON in big, bold letters — at the gate, as if we were drivers picking up a celebrity.

Some Michael Jackson song was on the radio. Jade settled into her drive while I adjusted my seat, leaned back, and tried to relax.

I heard a clunk.

"My phone fell," Jade said. "Could you get it? It's on the floor on your side."

I adjusted my seat to its upright position and bent over to pick up the phone when the car suddenly came to a screeching halt. I will never forget the sound. It was the most devastating, metallic, soul-crushing sound I had ever heard. It was the sound of finality.

Then *everything* went black.

When I opened my eyes, I realized we had just been in an accident. I had no idea how, or why, or how long ago it had happened. We were inside the car, but it wasn't moving. Smoke was everywhere. Were we upside down or still on the road? Maybe the car was on fire! A million scenarios raced through my brain and screamed for me to react, all at once. My whole body felt numb.

Jade! Where was she? Was she...

I looked for her through the smoke. Although she was only inches away, in my dazed state, she may as well have been in another dimension.

"Jade! Are you okay?"

"Mom? I think my arm is broken."

Panicked and relieved at the same time, I remember starting to yell: "I have to get out, I have to get out, I have to get out!" frantically searching for the door handle.

"Mom!" I heard Jade say, and then everything went black again.

When I woke up, I realized that I was sitting on a dark, wet road and had no idea how I had gotten there.

My head hurt. *What was happening?*

The bright lights of an ambulance, fire trucks, and police cars lit up the night. Still in a daze, I saw firemen working to clean up the mess.

"Ma'am, can you stand up?" a young woman in a paramedic uniform asked.

"What?"

"You've been in an accident. Can you stand up?"

"I… think so," I said shakily.

As she helped me get up and led me over to the ambulance, I noticed the front of my SUV smashed like an accordion against the front of a much larger SUV.

Off to the side of the road, a young woman was crying hysterically.

"I am so sorry! I was lost and was just looking at my navigation on my phone for a second," she said to a policeman. "I didn't realize I had drifted into the other lane!"

I looked at the paramedic next to me. "Where's my daughter?"

"*She's right over there,*" *she said, pointing to a stretcher near the ambulance.* "*She's okay.*" My thoughts were jumbled. *Where are our purses and phones? Oh, no! Jon! Who will pick him up at the airport? I'm freezing. Did I remember to lock the coop before I left?*

"Sit down, ma'am," the young woman in an EMT uniform said, pointing toward the edge of the ambulance. "I need to check you for injuries."

"Mom!" I heard Jade call out. "Are you okay?"

I nodded. "Are you?"

"My arm hurts, but I'm fine."

After the EMT worker finished her exam, she helped me into the ambulance. As I sat there, several other people asked me lots of questions. I had trouble understanding them in all the chaos. They asked me for my signature on multiple papers. Still disoriented, I just signed them without knowing what they were.

"Our purses…" I asked.

"Right next to you," the EMT woman said.

I saw Jade being loaded onto the same ambulance as me on a stretcher, with a brace on her neck and a splint on her wrist.

"We need to call Adrianna, Mom."

"What? How? I don't know where my phone is."

"It's probably in your purse."

I reached for my purse and finally found it. I tried to focus on it but couldn't. The numbers were fuzzy.

"You better do it, hon," I said, reaching across the stretcher to put it in Jade's good hand. I felt pain in my shoulder and was dizzy.

I must have blacked out again because the next thing I remembered was that I was on a bed in a crowded hallway of a hospital emergency room.

I tried to remember how long I had been there. I had a blurred recollection of talking to a doctor. As I looked down the hallway, everything seemed funny — off somehow. When I looked to the left, I saw double.

Looking around, I was able to make out Jade on a stretcher a few yards down the hall, speaking with my sister-in-law, Gladys. *How did she know we were here?* I thought. *Where was Jon?*

I got off my hallway stretcher and had to hold onto it to get my balance before slowly weaving my way down the hall to Jade.

"Jade, honey, are you okay?"

"My wrist hurts."

"Chris, you should be lying down," Gladys said.

"I'm fine."

A thin, pasty-looking doctor, who appeared to be in a hurry, walked over to us.

"How's my daughter?" I asked.

"She's lucky," the doctor said. "It's only a sprain. Nothing's broken."

I was relieved.

Jade cried out when the doctor roughly slid a tight brace onto her wrist.

"That should help. Over-the-counter pain medication is fine. Just keep the brace on, and you should be fine in a few days." Then he left to attend to someone else.

"Is Jon here?" I asked.

"Jon just walked in with Mom," Gladys said.

"How…"

"I called Adrianna. She called Dad," Jade said.

"Then he called me and Mom from the airport," Gladys added. "Bob picked him up and drove him here."

Jon's brother was a good guy who was always there to help with anything.

Jon walked over a few moments later with my mother-in-law, Thelma.

"Thank God you're both okay. How are you feeling?"

"My wrist hurts. The doctor said nothing was broken," Jade said.

"That's good." He looked at me. "How are you feeling?"

"Not great. I'm dizzy and my shoulder hurts. When can we go home?"

"The doctor said they'll need to do a few more tests. If everything is okay, we can go home after that."

"Can someone make sure Adrianna knows we're fine?"

"I talked to her," Jon said. "She wanted to come home right away, but I told her you all were okay and that I'd keep her in the loop. She'll be here next weekend as planned."

"Thanks."

It took another few hours. Once the tests were done, we were ready to go. My dizziness and double vision were noted in the medical report, but no cause was cited. Other than that, they told us we were just banged up a bit. The paperwork contained the legally required statement that we should follow up with our family doctor in a few days. The nurse asked me to sign some papers. I had a hard time focusing on the paperwork, so I just signed them, desperate to get out of there and back home.

It was late when we got back, and my head hurt. Jade was in pain, so she took some ibuprofen. After helping her gingerly crawl into bed, I covered her up like I did when she was little.

"Thanks, Mom."

She closed her eyes. For a moment, I was transported back in time, watching my three-year-old finally give in to sleep.

"I feel so exhausted. My legs feel like lead weights, and my entire body hurts!" I told Jon as I climbed into bed.

"Well, you were just in a car accident."

"I wonder why I hadn't noticed all these aches and pains earlier in the hospital."

"You were still in shock. Thank God both of you don't have more serious injuries."

As I lay in bed, trying to absorb the events that had unfolded that evening, I couldn't stop thinking about that horrible sound. Why could I not remember the crash, but still feel the sound? The entire evening seemed like a blur as Jon turned the lights out and got into bed.

I woke up later than usual the next morning, stiff and sore with a dull headache. After a quick shower, I exhaustedly sat down at the breakfast table. Jon and Jade were already there.

"How do you feel?" Jon asked, pouring me a cup of coffee.

"Not great. A little achy. I'm still seeing double. It's really weird."

"You're still woozy."

"Probably. How are you doing, hon?" I asked Jade.

"My arm really hurts. I know they said it wasn't broken. I've had broken bones before, and this feels the same."

"Give it time," Jon said.

"I guess. At least we're here to complain about it."

"Yeah, it could have been worse," I agreed. "We were lucky."

"Did you take a good look at both cars?" Jon asked.

"I recall seeing them all smashed up. It's kind of a blur."

"Same here," Jade said.

"I want to go to the tow lot today to view the damage."

"I want to come too!" Jade said.

"Are you sure you're feeling good enough?" I asked her.

"Yes. I feel bad, but it won't take too long. I really would like to go. Maybe it will get my mind off my arm pain."

"Damn, I have a hair appointment in a few hours," I remembered.

"Do you think that's a good idea? Driving might be hard right now," Jon said.

"Well, I'm pretty sure I can drive. It's only a two-minute drive down the road. It's hard to get an appointment on Saturdays," I answered as I gazed around the room, perplexed at the way things looked.

"Okay, if you're sure."

"I think it'll be fine. The doctors said I was just banged up. They would have told me if I shouldn't be driving."

"Then Jade and I will go to the tow lot while you're at your hair appointment."

"Wait, I have no car!" I exclaimed. "I just realized that!"

"Take mine," Jade said.

After Jon and Jade left for the tow lot in his truck, I got into Jade's car. As I adjusted the mirrors, I felt a sharp pain in my left shoulder that I hadn't noticed earlier. I realized my vision was double when I looked to the left, and I felt weirdly off. *Maybe I shouldn't be driving after all?* I went back inside the house. My hair would have to wait.

Jon and Jade got back a few hours later to report that our brand-new car was totaled.

"Are you sure?"

"Yep. It's a wreck. The garage guy agreed."

Jade looked at me. "No hair appointment?"

"No. My shoulder hurts, and my vision is double when I look in certain directions. It seems okay — maybe a little off — when I look straight ahead. I can't describe it."

"Good move. You need to rest up, Mom."

"I'll call the insurance company to get an assessor down to look at the car. Maybe we'll get something back."

After an early dinner, Jon went outside to take care of the coop. Jade and I tried to play a board game. I was having trouble concentrating, so we turned on the TV instead. No luck with that either, as I couldn't see the screen clearly. We went up to take naps. Jon made dinner, but neither of us had much of an appetite.

It is safe here in this darkness,

And scary on that stage,

But I move my chair a little closer,

To catch a glimpse of those who have engaged.

CHAPTER 6

The next day, Jade and I woke up with more aches and pains than the day before. We both had pounding headaches. My vision hadn't improved, and my shoulder hurt so much that I was barely able to lift the coffee pot. Jade couldn't even butter her toast.

Jon looked at us both. "Tomorrow, I'm calling Dr. Jeff."

Dr. Jeff had been our family doctor for years. He was always pleasant and had a fatherly manner. At the appointment, I noticed that his brown hair was now sprinkled with some gray. He examined Jade first. She winced when he touched her wrist.

"Did they do an X-ray in the ER?"

Jade shrugged. "I don't remember. They said it was just a sprain."

"With all this swelling, it looks broken. We'll have to take an X-ray to know for sure."

Then he examined my shoulder. I could hardly move my arm, and my neck was stiff and painful.

"How about you, Chris? Did they take an X-ray?"

"They did a bunch of tests. I'm not sure. It's all a blur."

"Okay. I think you both have more serious injuries than the ER said. I'm referring you both to an orthopedist I know. He's got the equipment in his office. I'll call him to get you in as soon as possible. I think Jade's wrist might be fractured, you have a shoulder injury, and both of you have whiplash."

"What about our headaches and my double vision?" I asked.

"Well, from what you told me about the crash, you both probably suffered concussions. Did they mention it to you or do any tests?"

"Again, I can't remember."

He shook his head. "ERs are too busy to be as thorough as they need to be. That's why it's always good to follow up with a family doctor."

"Could the concussion be why I see double?"

"Maybe. Vision problems often follow concussions."

He had me focus on his finger as he moved it right to left and back again.

"Looks like your eyes are having trouble moving left and right. It should improve over time. Don't strain your eyes by reading too much."

I nodded.

"Jade, how's your vision?"

"Fine. Just headaches."

"You both will need at least two weeks off work to recover, and no driving until I approve it. Ask Beverly to make an appointment."

"Two weeks!" Jade said. "My boss won't like that. I have to work." She worked at a local fast-food place.

I felt the same way.

"You've both been through serious trauma. You need time. I'll write you both medical notes for work. I'll see you both again in a few weeks after you see the orthopedist."

When we got home, we both called our bosses. Jade's was surprisingly understanding. While mine was cordial, I could hear the trepidation in his voice. There were no substitute teachers for my classes, and he knew my absence would place a burden on the already overworked technology department.

Jon took Jade to her scheduled appointment with the orthopedist for her wrist the next day. My appointment was a few days later. Normally, I would have insisted on taking her, but I wasn't allowed to drive.

When they returned, Jade was sporting a new soft cast and a neck brace.

"Well, my wrist *is* fractured. I don't know why the X-ray didn't show it in the ER."

I looked at Jon, who just shook his head.

"More oversights by the ER team. Thank God for Dr. Jeff."

"I also have whiplash and get to wear this cool neck brace for the next few weeks — and go to physical therapy."

I felt angry that Jade was misdiagnosed. What else would the specialist find for me when I *visit tomorrow?*

When we got to the orthopedist, Jon offered to come in with me.

"You should let me go in with you. I could ask questions and help."

"I don't know. I think it makes me feel like a little kid, like I'm not capable of doing it myself. Thanks anyway."

"I'll be in the car."

My visit to the orthopedist confirmed what Dr. Jeff had suspected. He examined me and took an X-ray.

"Looks like your rotator cuff might have been torn badly during the accident. You may need surgery," he said.

"Surgery? I thought it was just a bad bruise."

"We'll know more once you get an MRI. In the meantime, wear this sling." He helped me put it on.

My shoulder felt instant relief from the dull, constant ache. At the same time, the strap was killing my neck.

"Can we adjust it so it doesn't hurt my neck?" I asked. He tried, but my neck was so sensitive it still hurt.

"Sorry about that. Wear it when you go out of the house or when moving around a lot. Then take it off when you're sitting to rest your neck."

"Okay. What about my headaches and vision?"

"You may be suffering from the effects of whiplash and a concussion."

"Do I need a neck brace like my daughter?"

"I don't think it will help unless you have severe neck pain."

"No, I'm just a little stiff and sensitive."

"Then there's no need. My nurse will arrange for the MRI and make another appointment to review it."

When I returned to the car, Jon was on the phone.

"Okay, thank you," he said in exasperation as he hung up.

"What's going on?"

"That was the insurance assessor. The car is officially totaled."

"Great."

"What did the doctor say?"

"I need to get an MRI. The orthopedist thinks I tore my rotator cuff and might need surgery."

"What did he say about your neck?"

"Whiplash."

"Did he prescribe physical therapy like Jade?"

"No, I'm not in as much pain as she is. I think he was more concerned about my shoulder. He also said something about a concussion. I'm due back in a few weeks."

"Dr. Jeff was right again."

"Let's go home."

***

"You know, this accident was not our fault," Jon said later over dinner. "You said you heard the other woman admit it. I think we need to call a lawyer."

"How can a lawyer help?"

"I don't know. We need to do something. I'm not sure how this insurance thing works. Maybe there's a way to get reimbursed from the driver's insurance company for the car and all the time you and Jade are losing from work. You had to drop out of this semester's master's class. Pain and suffering too."

"You've got a point."

"Don't you know a guy from your class who became a lawyer in Philadelphia?"

"You mean Pat Anguilla? He's a divorce lawyer."

"He might know someone who does liability stuff."

"Okay, I'll call him."

Pat was helpful and gave me the name of a reputable personal injury lawyer he knew — Henry Ardsdale, based in Philadelphia.

Jon gave him a call and explained the situation. Henry said it sounded pretty straightforward and asked if he could meet with us at his office.

"We're about two hours away," Jon said. "Can we meet you halfway?"

We agreed to meet at a diner about half an hour from our house a few days later to discuss the case. He told us to bring all the medical documents we had and the police accident report.

***

Henry was waiting for us when we arrived. His handshake was firm, and his greeting was welcoming. I immediately felt comfortable. Over coffee, he went through all the documents.

"Your case is fairly cut and dried. The driver of the vehicle that hit you admitted to looking at her navigation on the phone she was holding in her hand while driving, which is illegal in this state. She admitted full responsibility."

As he went on to explain the legalities, I was having trouble concentrating. My vision doubled when I looked in certain directions and became slightly blurry when I looked in others. The sounds of the deep fryer alarms seemed ear-piercingly loud. The murmuring of the other diners didn't help. Since the accident, I had become increasingly sensitive to sound and background noise.

"I'm sorry, can you repeat that?" I asked.

"So, the bottom line is that we have grounds to sue for any damages that you've incurred."

I felt uncomfortable about this. I remembered seeing that poor woman weeping that night.

"I don't want to ruin that woman's life."

"You're not suing the driver, only her insurance company," Henry said. "The only thing that will happen to her is her rates will go up."

"What about our car insurance?" Jon asked.

"You pay insurance premiums, so you should be entitled to some compensation for expenses incurred from an accident by your company as well. I'll have to look at your policy to be sure."

"Will they cover medical bills and loss of work time?" Jon asked.

"They're considered part of the damages, depending upon your recovery time and medical expenses. Most insurance companies will fight you on the amounts you're owed. That's why you need legal representation."

"How long will all of this take?" I asked.

"Could be months, even a year or more. Insurance companies tend to string it out as long as possible."

"That's a long time," Jon said.

"It's my job to keep their feet to the fire. In the meantime, you need to document everything: doctor appointments, diagnoses, medical procedures, medications, lost time from work, and all other monetary expenditures and losses each week, and send them to me for the case file. Insurance companies usually settle, although there is a possibility that if they don't, we may need to go to trial."

"Trial? Really?" I said.

"That's the way it works. Usually, only cases with more extensive injuries go to trial."

"How much will this cost?" Jon quietly asked.

"Nothing until you get a settlement. Then I will get a percentage of that."

We asked him to give us a moment to discuss it. He left to make some calls.

"He seems to know his stuff," Jon said. "I think we should do it. It won't cost us anything unless we win."

My head was throbbing, and I just wanted to get out of there.

"Okay," I said.

Henry came back. "What did you decide?"

"We'll go for it."

"Yes, I think that's the way to go." He opened his briefcase and took out the representation agreements. Jon and I signed.

"I'll be in touch. Send me all your information. Call me anytime if you have any questions. Don't worry and feel better."

I was relieved to get out of that diner. Once in the car, I closed my eyes and tried to get comfortable for the ride home. I had the uneasy feeling that I was entering a new phase in my life and did not know what to expect.

"How did it go?" Jade asked when we got home.

"We're starting a lawsuit," Jon said.

"How long will it take?"

"Forever," I said. "I'm going to check on the coop."

I stood but felt a little wobbly.

"Mom, let me help."

"Thanks. I'll be fine."

***

The chickens gathered around me as soon as I walked into the yard. I struggled a little to fill the feeders and water containers, with my arm still in a sling. Despite the pain, I was happy to be with my flock again. Jon had taken care of them most days since the accident, and I missed them.

Feeling lightheaded, I decided to sit down on the grass. Everything seemed off, and I still couldn't figure out why. I could see directly in front of me, but to see anything around me, I had to move my eyes or my neck — both of which hurt.

While sitting on the cool ground to observe, as I had done many times before, I thought about how simple *their lives were. No doctors, no lawyers, no bosses. Just living day to day, doing the best they can.* I reminded myself of that simple goal. Despite all the challenges and distractions, my life now had one purpose: getting better. The rest was just a distraction.

Suddenly, Ruby ran over to me and jumped into my lap. A Rhodebar chicken with a full breast and deep reddish-colored feathers with fine buff barring on the edges, she was one of the three new hens we had obtained a few months ago. For some reason, she never seemed to fit in with the rest of the flock.

After years of observing, I found that chickens, like humans, have a hierarchy — a pecking order. Ruby was at the bottom of the pecking order and was relentlessly picked on. She knew I would protect her.

I would occasionally bring her into the house, where she would sit on a blanket for a while before happily exploring the kitchen and inspecting Riley and Daisy's bowls.

I bent over and took her into my arms, stroking her beautiful soft feathers. As I held her, I thought about chickens and their pecking order. I remembered reading that those at the bottom of the pecking order aren't sad. They accept whatever rank they are given and find happiness there. A chicken will be given many chances to fight for a higher status in the flock. Unless she takes advantage of those chances, she just settles in her place and is content. Like Ruby.

"Chickens are bitches!" Jon always reminded me when he saw me comforting Ruby.

That comment always made me chuckle.

Then, I thought about what our attorney had said about my being entitled to compensation after the accident. My first impulse was to simply accept my fate and not stand up for myself.

I thought about Ruby.

I refuse to be like her. I need to fight for what I deserve.

They laugh and cry, and love and die,

Upon that stage, exposed,

While I just sit here hiding,

Frozen in fear of the unknown.

CHAPTER 7

Over the next week, naps seemed to be my only escape from my vision issues, but I was tired and bored lounging around all day. When Adrianna came home for the weekend, and Jon, Jade, and Adrianna said they were going to the grocery store one afternoon, I eagerly tagged along.

It was my first trip to a store since the accident, and I immediately noticed the bright ceiling lights and the loud crackling music playing through the low-quality store speakers. *Weird — I've been going to this store for years and never noticed this.* I had become unusually sensitive to both light and noise since the accident.

I stopped to look at a display. I tilted my head to see the label clearly and then felt nauseous.

Looking up, I realized that Jade had gone down the aisle. I hurriedly walked to join her. Everything to the left was double, and everything straight ahead was slightly blurry. I was feeling a bit woozy.

"Chris?" said a voice behind me.

My chest tightened as I turned around. It was Velma, a fellow teacher.

"Velma… hi."

"How are you? I heard you were in a car accident."

"Yes, it was a few weeks ago. I'm doing okay."

"Glad to hear it. We miss you at school." She started to fill me in on the latest gossip.

I found it hard to concentrate on what she was saying, so I just nodded. *Why was it so hard to have a simple conversation in the store? I'd done it for years, bumping into neighbors and friends.* My head was pounding. I had to get away.

"Sorry, I have to catch up with my daughter. Great to see you. Talk soon." Trying not to stumble, I walked away, leaving Velma midsentence.

I walked toward Jade, only to pass her by.

"Mom, I'm over here. Are you okay?"

"Not really. Can we go home?"

"Sure. I'll find Dad."

I guess I still wasn't ready for prime time yet — even a place as familiar as the supermarket.

***

As the days passed, I felt as if my whole world had shifted. Everything looked different. *It had been two weeks since the accident. Shouldn't I feel better by now?* At some point, I realized that Jon and Jade had been taking care of the chickens without me asking them to. When Adrianna visited, she cleaned the house. The days all seemed to be blending into each other. *Why didn't I seem to care?*

Dr. Jeff called to see how I was doing. When I said my vision was still a problem, he suggested I try an eye patch on my left eye. Although it eliminated the double vision, it was scratchy and uncomfortable, and it greatly reduced my field of vision. It was not a viable solution, and I gave it up after a while.

I tried to relax by watching TV. It was frustrating because I had to tilt my head and try to sit at different distances and angles from the TV to avoid seeing double. When that didn't consistently work, I held a wooden spoon over one eye to prevent the double vision. That helped a lot, but eventually, my arm became tired.

I eventually figured out that if I sat in the exact spot on the couch where the TV across the room was slightly to my right and angled a certain way, I could finally enjoy a show. I also learned it helped to occasionally glance, not stare, at the screen while intently listening to the sound. Trying to relax was exhausting.

CHICKEN THERAPY

I was anxious to attend our two-week follow-up with Dr. Jeff. He was pleased with Jade's progress. Her arm was now cast and minimally painful. The physical therapy was helping her neck, and her headaches had eased.

However, my examination didn't go quite as well.

"Your concussion symptoms and double vision do not seem improved," Dr. Jeff said. "I recommend you see a neuropsychologist to evaluate you further."

"I thought you said it would improve with time. I don't think I need a psychologist."

"A neuropsychologist is not a psychotherapist. They specialize in brain-related injuries, including concussions. He'll be better able to find the best treatment for you."

"If you think it will help…"

"How's the shoulder?"

"It's a torn rotator cuff. I'm due to go back to the doctor next week. If I don't need surgery, I'm hoping to go back to work after that."

"Given your other symptoms, you might need more time before returning to a daily work schedule. I'll write a work excuse for another two weeks. The other doctors can extend it if needed."

I realized he was probably right. *How could I get back to work when I couldn't even focus on a computer screen at home?* I was worried. "I'm not sure I can afford to take more time off. I'm already out of sick days."

"I know, but you don't want to jeopardize your recovery by going back too soon. You may want to inquire about short-term disability. Most employment policies will cover you after ten missed days."

"Thanks. I never had this kind of problem. I'll look into it."

"Good. Let me know if I can help. Be sure to have the other specialists send me your reports."

I left the office feeling defeated. It sounded like there was no end in sight to my problems.

Jade could tell I was upset. "Don't worry, Mom. You'll get over it sooner than you think."

Uncle Bob was waiting in the car. He had been kind enough to drive us.

"How'd it go?" he asked.

"I'm getting better," Jade said.

"No change for me," I said, trying not to cry. "More doctors. More time off from work."

"Sorry about that."

"Yeah, me too."

That night after dinner, I shared the news from Dr. Jeff with Jon.

"Sounds like you need to check your teaching contract about short-term disability insurance," he said.

"Why? I might be better after I see the neuropsychologist."

"Couldn't hurt."

I got angry. "Don't you think I'll ever get better?"

"Sure I do. It's just that we need to be realistic. Your symptoms are still there."

"Meaning what?"

"You forget things, you can't do more than one thing at a time, you don't want to make phone calls or see friends. You say it hurts your brain to pay bills or think about anything remotely complex. You're pretty miserable."

"That is an exaggeration!" I snapped.

"And you're mad a lot."

"Wouldn't you be?"

"Yes, and you're taking it out on me. I've been trying to help as much as I can."

"You just don't get it!" I shouted as I turned and went upstairs. *Damn, I just yelled at Jon. What is happening to me?*

I got ready for bed and, exhausted, fell asleep quickly. I didn't hear Jon come in.

***

The next day, I called HR at the school and informed them about my situation.

"Chris, you do know that you're out of sick days, right?" Sally, the head of HR, said.

"I know. I thought I'd be back to work by now. It's going to take longer than I expected. What is the policy on short-term disability?"

"Well, you certainly qualify. I'll send you the paperwork. Since you'll be out on an undetermined leave of absence, your health insurance premiums will come out of your disability stipend."

"Could you tell me what the amount would be?"

"It's usually about half your usual salary, minus the insurance. I'll have to figure it out, and I'll get back to you."

"When will it start?"

"Probably in two weeks after you sign the paperwork."

"Okay, thanks."

I hung up and started to panic. How will *we* be able to survive without my full salary, especially now with all the out-of-pocket medical expenses?

That night, I told Jon about my conversation.

"How are we going to make ends meet?"

"Well, at least you'll have some money coming in. We can try to cut back on some things and use the credit cards if necessary. We'll get by — we always do. Hopefully, we'll get enough from the settlement to pay off any new debts."

"Who knows when, or what amount, if any, we'll get."

"I can start looking for a new job, one with paid health insurance. It'll work out. Don't worry — just relax and concentrate on getting better."

Jon never needed to get a job with good benefits before, because in the past, my teaching job had supplied them.

"I guess. Sorry for all this."

"We'll be fine," he said, taking my hand.

I am drowning in this ocean,

Being tossed and turned by the waves, at their will,

The more I fight against this force of nature,

The more the ocean proclaims its power over me until…

CHAPTER 8

Adrianna called daily to chat. Jade still lived at home, and I was thankful to have her around again. She could now help around the house and with the flock. On the days Jade and I were home alone, I would try to enjoy binge-watching TV with her. Despite my workarounds, I still had problems seeing the TV, but it was fun sharing time with her.

One of the people I relied on to drive me to my appointments was my 80-year-old father. Despite our relationship having had its ups and downs over the years, I was thankful for this opportunity to spend time together. I couldn't help feeling embarrassed that my father had to drive me around as if I were a teenager again, though.

"Where to today?" he asked one morning.

"The neuropsychologist," I said, giving him the address.

"What is that?"

"I'm not sure. It has something to do with my concussion. Dr. Jeff recommended I make the appointment."

"Well, I guess if Jeff thinks it will help."

We pulled into the parking lot of a large, modern building.

"You want company?"

"No, thanks."

"Okay. I'll be here."

I walked up to the main entrance and tensed up when I noticed there was a revolving glass door. Before the accident, I had no problem with revolving doors. Now, I found it hard to judge when it was the right time to step in. I waited until no one else was entering, took a deep breath, and stepped in. I had to go through a full rotation before nearly stumbling out of the doors into the lobby, feeling nauseous and sweaty.

I made my way to the reception desk.

"Can I help you?" the receptionist asked.

"I've got an appointment with Dr. Sharon."

"Name?"

"Chris Helm."

The receptionist checked his computer screen. "Yes, she's on the fourth floor. The elevator is to your left."

I hesitated. *Left. That was my double vision side.* As I looked left, everything was blurry and doubled.

"Are you okay, ma'am?"

I just nodded and slowly headed in the direction of the elevator. I was dizzy but made it. Luckily, a woman followed me inside as the door opened.

"What floor?" she asked.

"Four, thanks." I was grateful not to have to try to find the right button.

Why was I so anxious about doing such a simple thing as finding an elevator button?

Thankfully, the entrance to the doctor's office was directly in front of the elevator, so I got out and walked right in.

"Yes?" the doctor's receptionist said curtly.

"I'm Chris Helm. I've got an appointment with…"

She checked her screen. "At eleven. The doctor is running a bit behind. Please take a seat. I'll call you when it's time."

"Okay, thanks."

As usual, I had to fill out several forms that made my eyes hurt, then waited longer than expected.

"Chris Helm," an assistant said, escorting me into Dr. Sharon's office. Her office space was dark, dreary, and windowless.

Dr. Sharon stood up behind her desk and greeted me politely. She was pregnant. "Hi, I'm Dr. Sharon."

"Chris Helm."

CHICKEN THERAPY

The smartly dressed young doctor sat at her desk, invited me to sit opposite her, and then opened a file.

"I see you're here because of vision issues related to a concussion sustained in a car accident."

"Yes."

"We'll begin with a short questionnaire to get a baseline. Are you familiar with computers?"

"Yes."

"Okay. It will take about ten minutes. Can you manage that?"

"I think so. Sometimes it's hard to…"

She didn't let me finish. "Good. The computer is on the desk behind you. Just press enter and follow the prompts. I'll be back in a few minutes."

The type on the screen was small, and I had to concentrate hard to read it. Each question asked me to rate a range of symptoms such as dizziness, nausea, sensitivity to light and dark, sound, double vision, and headaches on a scale of 1 to 10. After a few minutes of looking at the computer screen, my head and eyes hurt. I could not complete the questionnaire.

"Finished?" Dr. Sharon asked as she came back.

"Sorry, I couldn't finish. My eyes and head began to hurt."

"Oh, I'm sorry," she said, somewhat surprised. "I'll ask you the questions verbally. Answer as best you can."

"I appreciate it."

"Are you sensitive to light?"

"Yes, very."

"Are you sensitive to noise?"

"Yes, mostly in restaurants and stores."

"Do you often feel lightheaded?"

"Sometimes."

"Okay. Please stand up, close your eyes, and try to stand on one leg. I'll be here to make sure you don't fall."

I stood, bent one leg, and immediately started to sway. She caught me.

"Well, that didn't go well," I said cheerily, trying to cover up my embarrassment.

"No worries." She then asked me to count backward from 20. When I passed 0 and continued counting into the negative numbers, she interrupted me.

"Um… that's fine."

I felt bad for attempting to be a smart ass and annoyed at myself.

"I'm going to say five words, and then you repeat them back to me. Ready?"

"Yes."

"Giraffe, table, pants, sky, and house."

This will be a piece of cake.

"Giraffe, table—" I quickly repeated.

Suddenly, I couldn't remember the next word.

"House… there's one before that… I don't know."

The next question involved listing five words that begin with a particular letter. The first time was the letter "F." Although I tried desperately to think of five words, the only one that came to mind was "fuck."

"Sorry…"

"Don't worry. That happens to a lot of people."

At the end of the session, she tallied up a score based on my responses.

"You've displayed symptoms linked to a concussion."

Duh.

"We should begin therapy immediately. I'd like to see you back weekly for a month. I'd also like you to see my colleague, Dr. Barrett, for concussion therapy twice a week. You can make the appointments at the desk."

"How will all this help with my double vision?"

"We hope to assist you in lessening the symptoms."

"Will it cure my issues?"

"I'm afraid it's too soon to tell. We'll need to wait and see." She stood. "Nice to meet you. I'll see you next week."

More doctor appointments. That's what my life had become.

I arranged the appointments and left.

After struggling with the elevator and revolving doors, I walked to my father, who was waiting in his van, reading the paper.

"I am so sick of all of this!" I said angrily, slamming the door.

"What happened?"

"Nothing. Just more appointments. And the worst thing is that she couldn't tell me whether any of it would cure me."

"Take some advice from your old dad. Doctors are there to help. They don't know everything. Give it a chance, and if it isn't helping, you don't have to keep going."

"Okay. Thanks, Dad."

"How'd it go at the neuro-shrink?" Jon asked when he got home, trying to add a little humor to my situation.

I told him about the experience.

"I guess all you can do is follow the therapy and see how it goes."

"I guess." I rubbed my shoulder.

"Still hurting?"

"Yep. I see the orthopedist next week. More fun."

Just before sundown that evening, I bundled up for the February cold and retreated to the coop to tend to the flock. After gingerly filling the feeder and checking the water, I felt a bit woozy and took a seat on the frozen grassy hill near the coop to enjoy watching the chickens and ducks milling about before shooing them inside.

Queen Elizabeth was always first in line to eat the dried mealworms. She was at the very top of the pecking order and pushed the others around like an entitled diva. Everyone else knew to toe the line. Ruby trotted toward me, knowing she was safe from the Queen and others if she stayed close to me.

Suddenly, Concussion Chicken raced over and stole a worm out of my hand, causing a few chickens to pursue her. She earned her name a few years ago when Jade had accidentally dropped a loose plank on her while helping in the coop. She flopped over on her side, and we were afraid she was dead. We were thrilled when she suddenly perked up and started to walk dizzily around. Ever since, she always wandered around the yard as though she was lost.

I shook my head as she tried to escape with her worm, swaying from side to side. Watching her stumble around, trying to avoid the other chickens, I had a sobering thought:

What if I never recover from my concussion like her? Will I be stumbling through life?

***

The following week, Jon drove me back to the orthopedist.

After waiting for half an hour, I was taken into an examination room. I waited another fifteen minutes.

"Hi, sorry for the delay," Dr. Gerald said as he walked in.

He checked my chart and examined my shoulder and neck. "Based on the MRI, you've got a serious rotator cuff tear in your shoulder. Your neck pain is the result of a herniated disc, but it's not serious. You'll need surgery for your shoulder, followed by physical therapy. The physical therapy should help with your neck as well."

"How long will the recovery from the surgery take?"

"Shoulder surgery is complicated. I would say anywhere from four to eight weeks, not counting the physical therapy afterward. The neck pain should get better after about a month." He glanced at my chart again. "You suffered a concussion also?"

CHICKEN THERAPY

"Yes. I'm going to therapy for it."

"You should be aware that the anesthetic used in the surgery could cause a delay in your recovery from the concussion as well. You need to discuss it with your doctor."

Great. More issues.

"How soon do I need the surgery?"

"That's up to you. The longer you wait, the more serious the tear might become. I advise that you schedule it as soon as possible."

As I left the office, I could feel sobs welling up from deep inside. I stumbled into the nearest bathroom, went into a stall, collapsed onto the edge of the toilet seat, and cried. I was so overwhelmed with it all.

"You okay?" Jon asked as I got into the car.

"No. He says I'll need surgery. The recovery will take months, and it will probably affect my concussion recovery. It's just endless."

"One step at a time. We'll get there."

I wasn't sure I shared his optimism about the future.

I decide to stop resisting,

Just drift into a sea of change.

Should I let the ocean win?

When bowing down feels so strange.

CHAPTER 9

The hardest part of my life after the accident was how the small, everyday things I always took for granted had become so problematic.

Like getting my hair styled.

Having to juggle all the doctor's visits, I finally managed to squeeze in my long-delayed hair appointment at my usual salon. I usually enjoyed getting my hair done while chatting with Linda, my long-time stylist. This time, it was a nightmare.

The place was busy as usual. As soon as I walked in, the sound of the buzzing hair dryers and the loud chatter of customers and stylists made me pause. Even though it was the usual situation at the salon, it made me nervous. I almost walked out but decided to go through with it.

"Hi, Chris," Linda said. "Glad you could make it."

I smiled. "Good to see you."

I sat down to have my hair washed, tipping my head back over the sink as usual. When the girl touched my head after wetting it, I jumped.

"Sorry," she said.

"That's okay."

The same thing happened when Linda began work. As soon as she touched my head, I pulled away.

"Chris, are you okay?"

"Sorry, I guess I'm still a little sensitive from the accident."

"Okay. I'll be quick."

I had to grit my teeth as she combed and cut my hair because my scalp hurt. I started to get a headache.

The young daughter of the owner was helping out by sweeping the cut hair on the floor. She was short, and the broom was too big for her. It banged into a chair next to mine on the left. As she came near me, I couldn't see how close she was and was afraid she might slip and hit my head with the broom.

"Do you mind having her not sweep around the chair until we're done?" I timidly asked Linda.

"Uh… sure," Linda said, asking the girl to move away.

The next problem was the noise. I thought I'd get used to it once I was in the chair, but I found it worse.

As soon as Linda finished the cut, I began to get out of the chair.

"I still have to do the color."

I knew sitting under the hair dryer would be torture.

"That's okay. I'll do it next time." I paid and got out of there as quickly as possible.

Then there was the simple act of getting fast food takeout.

On the way home from one of my doctor visits, Jon and I passed a new Mexican fast-food restaurant that had recently opened.

"Are you hungry?" I asked Jon. "I want to try this place."

"Sure!" he replied, pulling into the parking lot. "You wait here, and I'll go."

"No. I'll go in. What do you want?"

"I'll have what you're having."

I grabbed my purse and slowly stepped down from the truck. I steadied myself. *Get a hold of yourself. You can do this.* I shut the door and walked across the parking lot, looking straight ahead.

Once inside, I wasn't sure where to stand to order. Everything was blurry. The signs were awkwardly placed and hard for me to read. The noise from the busy lunch crowd didn't help. I just joined the line leading to the register.

I tried to figure out the lighted menu over the counter. The choices on the screen were doubled, and the details under the photos of each option were difficult for me to process. Luckily, the numbers next to each item were big and bold.

Suddenly, it was my turn.

"How can I help you?" the young man behind the counter asked.

I wasn't ready to order. Sensing the line behind me, I just blurted out, "I'll have two orders of number 3." I hoped it was something we liked.

"That will be $21.21, ma'am."

Opening my purse, it took me a while to find my wallet. When I opened it, there was a large wad of bills — a ten, a five, and a lot of ones. I tried to count out the exact amount but couldn't make out the denominations. I gave up and just put the wad on the counter.

The young clerk looked surprised, counted out $21, and gave me back the rest.

"Do you have 21 cents?"

"I think so." I fumbled for the change in my wallet, but I couldn't distinguish between the various coins. Frustrated, I just gave him another dollar. "Keep the change."

"Thanks." He handed me the receipt and two cups. "Your number is 53. We'll call you when it's ready. The soda machine is in the back."

I panicked. With all the background noise, I was afraid I wouldn't hear my number. I stood close to the counter to make sure. After receiving the order, I tried to navigate the maze of tables to the soda machine. My double vision made me feel disoriented and dizzy. I gave up and finally headed toward what I thought was an exit. It was the bathroom. I looked around nervously, found the exit, and left.

Barely avoiding a car backing out of a space, I got back to the truck.

CHICKEN THERAPY

"What took so long?" Jon asked as I opened the door and slid inside.

"Super crowded," I said quickly. I handed him the food.

"No drinks?"

"Sorry. The line was so long. I couldn't…"

"That's okay. I'll grab us something at the 7-Eleven next door. You start."

After he got out, I broke down. I felt weak and incompetent even doing the most routine things.

***

Anita, my concussion therapist, was always so supportive. When I shared my daily struggles with her, she was understanding. She explained that my experiences were normal following a concussion.

"You need to pace yourself, avoid any stressful situations, and get plenty of rest."

We would do simple exercises, such as walking the length of the sunny, cheerful room while counting backward from twenty. I was surprised by how difficult it was for me to do these simple multitasking exercises. Multitasking had always been one of my greatest strengths.

She also helped me understand more about my vision issues. "Your brain is having difficulty focusing on something near and then something far. That's why things sometimes seem blurry, and your eyes hurt."

"Is there anything I can do to help it?"

"I want you to practice at home for a few minutes at a time, looking at the writing on a can and then at something across the room. Then do it again a few times. If you start feeling bad, stop, close your eyes for a minute, and then try again. Don't push yourself."

Her advice was always spot-on and helped me cope with my challenges.

CHICKEN THERAPY

Unlike my sessions with Anita, my appointments with Dr. Sharon were depressing and exhausting. They made me feel like I was a case study instead of a patient. I dreaded the computerized tests she required. At the beginning of each session, I still had to rate my symptoms on the computer. I could never remember which number I had chosen at the last session, so I had no idea if I was getting better. I felt angry and depressed after each one.

Near the end of my time with her, she recommended that I see an ophthalmologist.

"What is that?" I asked.

"A physician who specializes in medical conditions affecting the eyes. Double vision associated with a concussion is normally gone by now. Since yours is not responding to therapy, it may be something physiological."

Yet another specialist. I tried to quell the feeling of panic that was overtaking my body.

"It sounds serious."

"It needs to be evaluated."

"Can I wait until after my shoulder surgery in two weeks?"

"I wouldn't. It's best to get the initial examination done so you can plan any future treatment. It's up to you, of course. I'll give you a referral." *Another trip down the rabbit hole.*

I shared this with Dr. Jeff, who thought it was a good idea. I made an appointment with an ophthalmologist, Dr. Carrie, a few days later.

Dr. Carrie was a well-dressed brunette who appeared to be in her late thirties. After introducing herself, she performed the usual vision tests I was familiar with from when I had gotten my contacts. This time, I could hardly read the eye chart because it was so blurry.

When she asked me to cover each eye and look at an object across the room, the image of the object seemed to jump around differently for each eye. She then had me follow her flashlight with my eyes. That hurt.

"It looks like you have some fourth cranial nerve injury to your right eye. That eye is not tracking correctly, and that is why you have double vision."

"You mean my nerve was damaged from the concussion?"

"Most likely."

"Is it permanent?"

"Hard to say at this point. You will need to see a neuro-ophthalmologist who specializes in eye problems related to nerve damage."

I sighed.

"There is only one in the area. My receptionist will give you the information. Good luck."

I felt like a ping pong ball, bounced from one specialist to another. Why couldn't anyone tell me what I needed to do to get back to normal?

I was beginning to wonder if anybody could help me. I called and made an appointment with the neuro-ophthalmologist for about a month after my shoulder surgery was scheduled.

As usual, my flock was my saving grace. Later that day, as I went out to the coop, I noticed most of the hens and ducks huddled under a bush near the coop. Ike was sitting alone on the edge of the hill. Suddenly, I saw a large hawk fly off over the hill.

Fearing the worst, I ran over to Ike, who appeared unharmed at first. He was just standing there. As I sat beside him, I noticed his labored breathing. Gently pushing aside his feathers, I inspected his body. Usually, he didn't like being touched, but this time he didn't budge. After finding numerous puncture wounds and some bleeding, I gently pushed him to see if he could walk.

He tried, then stumbled, heroically trying to move. That's when I knew his injuries were serious and that he was in pain. I gently picked him up, kissed him, and told him he had been a wonderful rooster.

CHICKEN THERAPY

Jon saw me and came over.

"Ike is in bad shape," I said. "I'm pretty sure a hawk got him."

"Poor guy."

We had been through this kind of predator attack a few times over the years. Early on, we had taken a few injured birds to the vet. It didn't take long to figure out that the chickens and ducks did not respond well to vet care, and the bills for these "specialty animals" were enormous. Jon and I created a humane way of handling this problem.

If we deemed a bird to be too ill or injured to survive, Jon would cull it from the flock and take it into the woods. I never knew exactly what he did after that. Jon always assured me that he was kind and humane.

Jon got a box, and then gently took Ike from me. As he placed him inside, Ike scuffled a bit, trying to regain his freedom. Thankfully, he quickly succumbed as Jon shut the lid. As he walked toward the woods, I shooed the rest of the flock back into the coop.

Despite his bravery, Ike had been in the wrong place at the wrong time. After his skirmish with the hawk, he valiantly tried to maintain his composure in the face of his injuries, trying to survive. Unfortunately, they proved too serious to overcome.

I tearfully lingered outside the coop so Jon wouldn't see my sadness when he returned. We had discussed many times the risks of letting the flock free-range outside the protected run. It was still hard when nature took its course. I was thankful Jon was brave enough to prevent any prolonged suffering.

I thought about my situation. Like Ike, I was the victim of an unexpected incident. We both fought to survive our trauma. Mine was difficult. It was not fatal. Ike's time was up. Mine was not. Realizing the finiteness of my life, I vowed to find a way to not only heal but to thrive.

I am so exhausted,

I have lost my will to fight,

My body can only float along,

While my eyes take in the sights.

CHAPTER 10

I finally had shoulder surgery. While it went well, as predicted, it affected the symptoms of my concussion. Even after the anesthesia wore off, my world became foggier. My double vision and dizziness got worse. The prescription painkillers to help with the surgical pain only added to it. There seemed to be no escape from my misery. No position — sitting, standing, or lying down — brought relief. Even sleep was a problem.

A week later, I started physical therapy. Even though it was painful and exhausting, the therapist was kind and friendly. The last 15 minutes of each session were always relaxing because I got to lie on a table with either heat or ice on my shoulder.

When I stared at the ceiling, the lines separating the tiles would be doubled, slanted, or blurred no matter how hard I tried to make them come into focus. I learned to always shut my eyes so I could enjoy the peaceful completion of the session.

The weeks flew by like a hazy dream. I seemed to be living in a strange new world, so unlike the one I had known. For the first time in my life, I had no busy daily schedule to keep.

Adrianna came home most weekends to help around the house and with the coop. She always left enough food and water for the ducks and chickens in case Jade and I weren't up to the task.

I kept a list of things like doctors' appointments, expenses, and symptoms on the kitchen counter. Every two weeks, Jade would scan any new documents and then email them to Henry, our attorney. Although the headaches, dizziness, and nausea were improving, I found that everything involving reading, typing, or using a computer was still very difficult.

I tried not to think too much about our finances. Bill paying had always been my job, and I insisted on holding on to that responsibility. Luckily, I had set up a system a while back for most bills to be automatically deducted from our bank account. It was a great help during my recovery because it required minimal reading or computer work. Over time, I recovered enough from the surgery to do some minor chores. When he was home, Jon pitched in as well. I was grateful for all the help but still felt a bit useless.

"I think Ruby has a cold," Jade said one day in early March after she came in from feeding the flock. "She's sneezing a lot. Time for rehab."

When a chicken or duck showed any signs of illness or injury, we would separate them by putting them in a large dog crate on the porch. In the winter, we had to keep them in a crate in the dining room, which we rarely used as we ate in the kitchen. The local feed store carried antibiotics and first aid supplies needed for general bird illnesses.

"I can set up the crate," Jade offered.

"Okay. I'll get her."

Ruby had become my favorite chicken in the flock. She was submissive and friendly. She followed me around the yard like I was her protector. Her constant soft clucks and curiosity about what I was doing when I was nearby always made me smile. She was always happy to see me and would even follow me into the house. I threw a bit of meal into the crate, and she walked right in.

"Now you guys can recoup together," Jade said, smiling.

If only it was that easy, I thought.

***

I tried to keep my immediate family and a few close friends updated about my ongoing progress. I had never been one to send group texts or post on social media. I always preferred to talk on the phone or meet in person. After the accident, though, everything about socializing seemed exhausting.

I had stopped accepting offers from worried family and friends who wanted me to "get out more." Most of my friends had given up on inviting me to gatherings. Even when I accepted an invitation, they all knew that I would inevitably cancel. A few steadfast childhood friends and fellow teachers still checked in frequently, though, and I was happy about that.

Dora, one of my closest friends, decided that she would no longer take no for an answer. "The next time Jon is away, I'm coming over and we are baking. No excuses."

I had known Dora since childhood and knew she wouldn't back down despite my protests. So, on Jon's next trip, we planned an early evening of baking. However, on that day, things had been challenging. I was tired and irritable, not up for company. I decided to cancel and left a message for her, saying that I had to postpone our date. I didn't hear back, so I assumed Dora would understand.

At the appointed time for our date, Dora came bursting through the back door, laden with a bag of groceries. I was eating dinner alone at the kitchen table.

"Dora, didn't you get my message?"

"Yes. I'm here anyway. Let's get started." She put the groceries on the counter.

"I'm not sure…"

"I've got all the ingredients. I'll read the recipe out loud, and we'll follow the directions together."

I laughed. "Team effort?"

"Right. You don't have to use your eyes if they're tired. You explain to me any parts I don't understand. You're the baker after all."

"True. You can't bake!"

"Where are your aprons?"

CHICKEN THERAPY

For the next few hours, we baked and chatted about our childhood memories and college antics. She didn't mention my vision issues or the accident. We were just good friends having a nice time. We ended up with dozens of chocolate chip cookies and lemon pound cake, which we sampled over coffee.

Later that evening, after she had left, I realized I had forgotten to close the run and the coop. After a quick head count, I shooed them into the coop and shut the door. I sat down inside the coop, relieved that all were accounted for. After exiting the coop, I lingered outside for a while, enjoying the night air.

Suddenly, I heard a loud shriek from inside the coop. I opened the door to find Ruby on the floor, squawking. She had tried to nudge her way in between Kevin and Queen Elizabeth. The Queen would have none of it and had shoved Ruby off the roost.

"Ruby," I said, picking her up, "you should know better." I lifted Ruby to the thick branch in the outcast roost in the corner of the coop. She quieted down.

Content that all was well for the night, I walked out of the coop toward the house and stood on the porch for a minute. I drew in a breath of the crisp night air, looked up at the sky, and wondered. *Had I created an outcast roost for myself by distancing myself from my friends?* I vowed to try harder to spend more time with good friends.

The next morning, I gazed out the window at the rapidly falling snow. Everything was covered in at least six inches of white, fluffy wonder, and the gray sky looked angry. Pennsylvania snowstorms can be fickle, especially the Nor'easters. When I was teaching, and the kids were little, I loved our "snow days" because that usually meant I could stay home and relax with them.

After folding a load of laundry, my shoulder ached. Even though I had mastered doing many activities with one arm, after a while my body just seemed to revolt. I decided that today I

CHICKEN THERAPY

wouldn't dwell on how I felt or think about doctors, lawsuits, or my recovery. My physical therapy had been canceled because of the snow. Today was a snow day — my day off.

I bundled myself up and wandered out to the chicken coop to check on my flock. Trudging up the hill, I found the chickens milling around inside the coop, except for Kevin, the young rooster who had inherited Ike's position. He was roosting by himself. *Odd*, I thought. Most chickens only roost at night. They perch as high above the ground as they can to be as far away from predators as possible while they sleep. They will only roost during the day if they feel threatened or sick.

Looking around, I noticed that Jon had cleaned the coop before he left in anticipation of the storm, knowing that the flock would probably spend a few days inside. I hated that he had to do that chore. That was always my job. To most people, cleaning a chicken coop seemed like a disgusting task. To me, it was weirdly fulfilling. I think it kept me grounded and grateful. It also reminded me that effort was always needed to reap the rewards of anything.

It was one of the many activities I missed — like teaching, driving, or meeting up with friends. They all were part of my independent life. I *need* to get back to that. Trying to keep despair from invading my thoughts, I focused on figuring out why Kevin was alone on the roost and stepped closer to examine him.

He seemed a bit sluggish and had black marks on his large, droopy comb. After examining it more closely, I realized it was frostbite. It had been below freezing that night after the snowstorm. He must have gotten his comb wet while drinking water, and it froze. I needed to put Vaseline on his comb to protect him from any further damage. First, I had to grab him to keep him still. I couldn't do it alone because of my shoulder.

I went inside to enlist Jade to help. We were able to corner Kevin long enough for me to coat his comb. We worked as a team, despite our injuries, to outwit the strong-willed but gentle rooster. Afterward, we rewarded ourselves with some of the cookies I'd baked and some hot tea.

****

In the spring, Jade had completely healed and was ready to return to work. To celebrate, Jon suggested we go out to dinner at one of our favorite places. It was a lively, pub-style restaurant in town that was always bustling and fun.

As soon as I walked in, the chatter of the patrons and the general commotion of the place hit me. It seemed so much louder than I remembered it being. My eyes started to hurt from the brightness of the lights. Regardless, I was determined not to spoil Jade's night.

Jon asked for a table in the back where it was a little quieter and less brightly lit. Even there, I could barely participate in the conversation because of the noise. I kept adjusting my position in my chair to see Jon and Jade without double vision. I felt like an outsider at my own family's celebratory dinner.

By the time the food came, I had lost my appetite. What was supposed to be a proud and happy moment had turned into an ordeal for me, and I was grateful to leave.

As I gaze into your eyes in the roller coaster line,

My world is complete, there is no meaning to time,

We step into the car, with our "us" still intact,

The coaster ascends, no need to react.

CHAPTER 11

The office of Dr. Brown, the neuro-ophthalmologist, was in one of several modern buildings on a large health campus. Jon insisted on walking with me into the building and waiting in the lobby. Normally, I would have been annoyed, but today, I felt grateful for his help with yet another revolving door.

After checking in, I had to fill out the usual sheaf of forms and wait. Fifteen minutes later, a nurse escorted me to a second waiting room. It seemed that most of the patients in this room were children, not adults. I thought that was strange.

When my name was called, a nurse brought me into an examination room. She verified my details and health profile and gave me what she called a pre-exam. She spent a lot of time moving objects in front of my eyes and watching how my eyes followed them. After writing down some notes, she directed me to return to the waiting room.

I dutifully returned to my place and waited. When it was finally my turn to see the doctor, I went into another exam room. Dr. Brown arrived, introduced himself, and looked at my file.

"I see you have some cranial nerve damage and double vision at times."

"Yes."

He had me cover one eye, look at an object far away, and then cover the other eye and look at the same object. The object seemed to jump around on the wall when I switched eyes, giving me that familiar unwell feeling. He then handed me a book. Its cover was black plastic, and its pages were stiff.

"Please take a look at the large fly on the first page."

"Okay. I see it."

CHICKEN THERAPY

"Does anything seem to pop out?"

"What do you mean?"

"Do the wings look like they pop out of the page?"

"I don't think so."

"Try the next page. There are six diamonds with circles inside. Do any of these figures or any of the circles pop out more than the others?"

"I don't think so."

"Try again more slowly, and be sure to focus."

I stared at the page for a moment longer, and suddenly, a circle popped out.

"Yes, that one." I pointed to it on the page.

"Great. Let's try the next page. Now look at the first row of animals. Does any one animal appear to pop out more than the others?"

By this point, I knew that one was probably supposed to look different, only it didn't.

"I'm sorry, I don't think so." I was getting frustrated. "What is the point of this test?"

"It is meant to gauge your ability to see in three dimensions and test your depth perception."

I didn't understand what viewing flat pictures had to do with either of those.

"So, how did I do?"

"Let's just say you are having difficulty with both. This test confirms that you've got a right fourth cranial nerve palsy. This nerve palsy can be more susceptible to damage because it is the only cranial nerve that starts at the back of the brain and has a longer path through the skull than any other cranial nerve. It enters the eye socket through an opening at the back and then travels to one of the external eye muscles."

"Is that what's causing the double vision?"

"Yes, and many of your other symptoms. This nerve controls the muscle that turns the eye inward and downward. So, when you look left to right, the image each eye sees does not currently line up in your brain. You have difficulty seeing three-dimensionally, and this affects your depth perception and coordination. Your brain is working very hard to compensate, and you feel the result."

"How bad is the damage?"

"Sometimes the nerve is only stretched and will bounce back with time and rest. There is the possibility that it may be permanently damaged."

"When will we know for sure?"

"Normally, after about six months. If your symptoms remain the same at that point, your nerve is considered damaged, not stretched. It is important to not push yourself to do any activities that make your eyes or brain tired at this point."

Six months!

"It's already been over three months since the accident. You mean it could take another three months before we know?"

"At least. I know it's frustrating, but you'll need to be patient. This kind of trauma takes time, especially as we age."

"Is there anything I can do to help with the symptoms?"

"Since your near- and farsightedness have not changed significantly, you can continue using your regular glasses."

"I usually wear contacts."

"It's the same. If you find reading is still blurry, you can supplement with generic readers from the drugstore. Just don't overdo it. We can re-evaluate your prescription if needed when things settle down. I'd like to see you in a month."

"What about returning to work?"

"What kind of work do you do?"

"I'm a math teacher and technology director. I spend a lot of time in front of computer screens."

"I'm afraid that it would not help your condition. I'd be happy to write you a work release for the next month. This is not something you can push through."

"Thanks," I said, knowing full well that my principal would not take kindly to this additional time off.

***

Over the next month, some of my concussion symptoms slowly improved. I could use the computer for ten to fifteen minutes without getting headaches. I practiced driving locally during the day. So long as there was no traffic and I stayed on familiar routes, I could manage short trips. We'd finally gotten another car—the same make and model—to replace the old one, so I was familiar with it.

Exercise helped clear my mind, get my blood flowing, and aid in my healing, so I continued to walk vigorously for an hour each day. I still attended PT twice a week for my shoulder.

The little things still plagued me. When I tried to write a to-do list, the words were blurry, even with the drugstore readers. When I tried to read the labels on groceries, I had to focus longer than usual. If the type was too small, I had to give up. Watching TV was still a challenge. While I tried to remain positive, these things ate away at me daily.

I tried to stay more in touch with friends, mostly by phone. While it was frustrating to listen to all the things they did in their busy lives that I couldn't even attempt, it was good to connect again. My friend Leslie called one day to invite me to our semi-regular girls' night out that Friday.

"It'll be great to have you with the old gang."

This would be the first time I had socialized with a group outside my family since the accident. I remembered that night of my dinner with Jade and cringed.

CHICKEN THERAPY

"I don't know."

"Come on. I'll pick you up. It'll be fun."

"Okay," I said, realizing I had to try to do something besides going to the store, going to doctor visits, and hanging out with my flock.

That Friday, I was anxious all day about the dinner. Lots of chatting in a loud, crowded restaurant, bright lights, double vision—it would be a lot to deal with. I was coping with my symptoms much better these days, so I hoped I wouldn't have the same experience I'd had with Jon and Jade at dinner a few months before.

I fixed my hair and put on one of my favorite outfits. It felt great to wear something other than leggings and a sweatshirt.

"You look terrific," Jon said, smiling.

"Thanks. I'm still nervous."

"You'll do fine. Everyone misses you. Have fun."

Leslie pulled up right on time. I got into the car, quickly buckled my seatbelt, and looked straight ahead without saying a word.

"Are you okay?"

"Sorry, I'm just a little anxious riding in a car with someone other than my family driving."

"No worries. I'll be super careful."

"Thanks for understanding."

On the drive to the restaurant, I tried to ignore the tight feeling in my chest as other cars got too close. We chatted about our lives and families, and I talked about my recovery efforts and, of course, the chickens. Leslie was so easy to talk to, and the trip seemed to go by in a flash.

It was nighttime, so walking from the car to the restaurant, I had to concentrate to keep my balance. The bright lights of the entrance hurt my eyes, but I tried to ignore them.

As soon as Leslie opened the door and we stepped inside, the laughter and conversations of the patrons in the packed restaurant immediately overwhelmed me. I felt panicked and wanted to leave.

"There they are."

She had spotted our other friends at a table on the side and waved before I had the chance to ask her to take me home. Instead, I followed her as she navigated the tables.

Upon approaching the table, I was dismayed that the table was long, not round, and that the only empty seats left were in the far corner. The only way I could see everybody would be to turn my head and look to the left. Having no idea how to articulate why I wanted to change seats, and not wanting to draw attention to myself, I just sat down and shifted my chair sideways.

Everyone was so friendly and welcoming. They ordered drinks. I stuck with iced tea.

"How are you feeling these days?" my friend Sara asked. It sounded as if she was shouting.

"Getting better."

"I'm glad."

Over dinner, it was difficult to keep up with my friends' conversations against all the background noise. I made out bits and pieces as they spoke of their vacations, their jobs, and their active lives. Compared to all their news, I felt as though I had nothing worthwhile to contribute and mostly sat there and smiled. I remembered that, at one of our earlier dinners, I had excitedly told them about my new position at school and that I was currently in a master's program. That seemed like ages ago. So much had changed since then.

As the evening wore on, my double vision and headache got worse. I had trouble concentrating on the conversation. I reverted to fake nods and chuckles to get through the evening. No one seemed to notice, and I was glad.

At the end of the evening, after standing up to leave, I looked around the crowded restaurant, searching for the restroom. I immediately felt disoriented and dizzy and stumbled slightly.

"Looks like someone had too much to drink tonight," Dora jokingly chided.

"I guess so," I said with a pretend giggle.

When we left the restaurant, Leslie offered to pull the car close to the entrance so I wouldn't need to walk through the lot.

"That's okay. I'd rather walk."

On the trip home, Leslie cheerily chatted about the evening.

"It's always nice to spend time with just the girls," she said.

"Yes, it was good to get out."

"We'll do it again soon."

Not likely, I said to myself.

"How was it?" Jon asked when I got home.

"Okay, I guess."

"That doesn't sound good."

"I guess I am not used to doing things in the evening. I'm exhausted."

"That is a shame. I was hoping that getting out would make you feel like your old self."

"My old self?" I snapped.

"You know what I mean."

I didn't want to admit that I knew what he meant.

"No. Enlighten me."

"I'm going to bed," he said.

After turning out the lights in the living room, I sat down on the sofa and softly cried. Lashing out at Jon was not something I used to do. It seemed that the harder I tried to get back to life before the accident, the further away it slipped.

***

The next day was warm and sunny. It was not quite spring, and the daylilies were peeping cautiously through the ground anyway. This was the kind of day that made me happy. I went out to tend my flock. The chickens and ducks were so excited to get out into the clean, fresh air. I opened the gate to let them roam free and hunt for bugs at the bottom of the hill while I cleaned up the coop.

I trudged to the top of the hill, took off my boots, and stood on the cool, fresh grass. Tilting my head to the left to avoid double vision, I noticed Ruby racing up the hill to greet me. I smiled and felt a moment of peace. I liked to think that she was coming to greet me, but I knew she was just looking for treats.

I could hear the crows calling from the trees, which usually meant a hawk was nearby. The chickens heard it too. A few more chickens followed Ruby's lead. They ran to me like combat soldiers, heads low, wings out, determined to get up the hill to me so I could protect them.

As they gathered around my feet, looking to me for protection, I felt comfort in the connection I had with them. They didn't see me as broken as I felt. They depended on me as they always had. It made me feel hopeful that I would be back to my old, independent life. It was spring, a time of rebirth. I desperately wanted a chance at a rebirth.

But, somehow on that trip up that steep hill,

A wheel came loose, and I was tossed will and nil,

I gathered my wits and looked all around,

The car was still climbing, but a part of me was on the ground.

CHAPTER 12

Jade drove me back to see Dr. Brown for my appointment. I didn't need to take any additional tests.

"How do you feel?" he asked.

"Not much has changed. My double vision is the same, although my other symptoms seem a little better."

He noted it in my file. "Sounds like you're still healing. Let's try a temporary prism sticker for your glasses to see if that helps."

"What is that?"

"They are clear stickers for glasses. They act as prisms that redirect the light to a place on your retina to help your brain fuse the double images. If the prisms are effective, then you may be able to return to work."

Finally, a ray of hope.

"I guess I'll need to give up my contacts." I disliked the way I looked in glasses and how they felt on my face.

"I'm afraid so. You can use your current prescription, though. With the new glasses, I don't think you'll need the readers anymore." He wrote the prescriptions out for me. "You can use the optometrist across the hall. I'll see you again in a month."

It sounded like it could work. Jade helped me pick out new frames. The optometrist said the glasses and prisms would be ready the next day.

Jade drove me to pick up the new glasses the following day. The prism sticker was a clear piece of plastic with barely visible slanted lines that covered one lens. I put them on and looked straight ahead.

"How do they feel?" the optometrist asked.

"I think I see more clearly. It kind of feels like what I see is delayed or something. It feels odd. I wish I could explain it!"

"It will take you a little time to get used to them. How about the double vision?"

I looked to the left. As I did, I felt a whirling sensation in my brain as the double images became less double, then blurry, and then went into focus as a single image.

"Oh, wow, while the double vision is better, it takes time to focus."

"It should get better as you get used to them. Good luck."

I walked out happy to see almost normally again. It was a minor miracle.

"The new glasses look great on you," Jade said. "How's the vision?"

"Much better. The prisms help with the double vision."

I wore the glasses every day afterward. The prism stickers improved my vision; however, as the day wore on, especially after driving, shopping, reading, or using the computer, even for short periods, eye fatigue, headaches, and nausea would set in, and my vision would regress.

Until that time, I could function pretty normally. I continued to regulate my activities, and I was grateful for even this breakthrough. I was sure that it would get better in time.

At my next appointment, Dr. Brown did a series of tests with me wearing the prism glasses. I found the tests much easier and accomplished many of the goals.

"The double vision seems to have stabilized with the prisms. How do you feel generally?"

"Much better. As long as I pace myself, I can read and use the computer almost as long as I used to. The headaches and nausea are better too, although my eyes get tired at the end of the day. I was able to drive here today on my own for the first time."

CHICKEN THERAPY

"That's great news. I think you should be able to go back to work, at least on a part-time basis initially, if you continue to feel better."

"You think so? Although I can't wait to get back, I am worried about my ability to keep up with the intensity of my job."

"I will send you to an occupational therapist who can help you navigate working with your lingering symptoms." He handed me a pamphlet about an agency. "I can give you a note to start back part-time. You can see how it goes. I will see you back in three months to see how things are going."

"Sounds good," I said, smiling. "Thank you so much."

On the drive home, I was worried. *Would the school agree to my returning part-time?* Teaching and being a technology integrator was a full-time job and then some. I was a little nervous that some of my symptoms might make work difficult, even part-time.

Once home, I immediately read the pamphlet. "Office of Vocational Rehabilitation (OVR) serves people with disabilities that present a substantial impediment to their employment. Services are provided to individuals who can benefit from and who need assistance to prepare for, enter, engage in, or retain employment."

With disabilities. That sounded like people who were permanently disabled. My concussion symptoms were getting better. So was my vision. If it meant getting back to work and my old life, I'd try it. I called the OVR and explained my condition.

"I have never heard of a case quite like yours," the pleasant woman who answered the call replied. "We normally deal with physical disabilities related to mobility or manual issues. Let me have one of our therapists give you a call back in a few minutes."

An hour or so later, the therapist called.

"Hi, I'm Brigitte Finch from OVR. I understand you're seeking occupational therapy because of vision issues related to a concussion."

"Yes. My doctor recommended this therapy to prepare me to get back to work. I'm a teacher." I explained the challenges with my double vision and other symptoms and how they might affect my work.

"I am not sure that regular in-person therapy sessions will be helpful for you at this point," she said after listening to me patiently. "But I can try to give you a few tips on the phone."

"I appreciate any help you can offer."

"Okay. You say that you still sometimes get a little dizzy when you stand up. Since you're a classroom teacher, I suggest standing up a few minutes before the class begins, and that way you can gather yourself beforehand. At meetings, you can do the same."

I realized that standing before a presentation would be helpful. On the other hand, when teaching, I frequently needed to sit down and stand up several times during class. I explained my concern.

"There's no one solution. If you need to get up from sitting, try to do it as gradually as you can."

"It might look a little weird to the students, but I'll try."

"You also said your eyes get tired as the day progresses and the double vision gets worse if you don't take a break. I suggest you set a timer and take a break every so often, maybe go to the bathroom and close your eyes for a few minutes."

"I wouldn't be able to do that during class or at meetings."

"Okay, then prepare yourself ahead of time as much as you can. Take a short break before and rest your eyes. Utilize your lunch time to rest."

As she continued with her suggestions, I realized that although she meant well, she truly had no idea what it was really like to be a teacher and a technology integrator. I was on call all day. Many days I would eat lunch in my classroom to accommodate the stream of students who used this time to seek my help.

I thanked her for the suggestions and hung up. I felt a tinge of anger and disappointment. Her "tips" weren't appropriate to my job. It looked like I was on my own. I had to make it work.

On the plus side, the timing was perfect. It was June, and the students were out of school. If I went back, I could work on the administrative needs of the tech program for a few hours a day, a few days a week, and slowly ease into the position before the fall and get ready to teach.

The next day, I called Sally in HR.

"I have been cleared to return to work part-time. I can run my doctor's release over to you later today," I excitedly said.

"Sounds good. I'll check with the principal, but it should be fine. I'll get the paperwork going. He'll give you a call."

Dr. Jeff had retired, so I made an appointment for a check-up with the woman who had taken over his practice, Dr. Lori McQueen. She was about my age and seemed professional, kind, and caring. I informed her about Dr. Brown's release to return to work part-time.

She looked through my file. "How are you feeling overall? Is your shoulder healed?"

I explained that I was nearing the end of my physical therapy treatments and feeling much better.

"How about your concussion symptoms?"

"The prism glasses have helped a lot. I still get some double vision if I read or use the computer for too long. Sometimes I have some difficulty with concentration. I also feel like I am not able to think as quickly as I used to. I am a little worried about that because teaching high school students can be demanding."

She informed me that a certain ADD (attention deficit disorder) medication was found to be very useful for people with post-concussion syndrome and asked if I was interested. She said it might help, especially with concentration.

Intent on doing anything that would make returning to work easier, I agreed to try it. She handed me a prescription and wished me luck.

The Vyvanse worked amazingly well. For the first few hours in the morning after taking it, I felt like my old, pre-concussion self. I was able to multitask and get things done more effectively. However, it wore off by early afternoon, and my concentration suffered. I had to be sensitive to the timing when I returned to work.

Adrianna came home and cooked us a celebratory seafood meal the weekend before my first scheduled day back to work.

"Here's to Mom's return to real life," she toasted before we ate.

As our glasses clinked, I felt a deep sense of love and gratitude for my family.

The part of me that was "us" seems so far away,

Even though I was still in that car beside you

on that same day.

CHAPTER 13

My first day went by quickly. Very few teachers were in the building because it was summer break. The administration and technology teams were the only staff members who remained in the building.

Without students, I could prepare for the upcoming school year at my own pace. I went in three days a week for a few hours in the morning. It allowed me to come home, take a two-hour nap, tend the flock, and do some chores around the house. I limited my reading and computer work.

Most days, I was able to manage my symptoms. I still felt slightly nauseous or dizzy if I stood up too quickly. I was still seeing double to some degree but was managing my job effectively despite these challenges. I was proud of my progress.

In mid-August, Jon came home and said, "Good news! I am scheduled to do a weeklong job at a beach resort in New Jersey next month. The hotel and meals will be paid for. Want to come along? The trip shouldn't cost us much more than gas."

I needed the break. I had gotten back to work and now was worried about how it would look to take a vacation.

"I'll have to check with the principal. It should be fine because I'm ahead of schedule for the preparations."

The principal approved. Jade took care of the flock and pets, so I went with Jon. It was the first vacation we'd had in years. I basked in the sun and swam in the ocean during the day while Jon was working. Jon and I dined at the lovely hotel restaurant and took long walks on the beach at night. It was like a second honeymoon. On the ride home from our getaway, I felt refreshed and energized.

My symptoms seemed to improve after our vacation. Over the next few weeks, I slowly increased my hours at school to work my way up to a five-day week in preparation for the beginning of the school year.

I soon recognized that although I was successfully doing my job, by the end of the day, I was exhausted. It was hard to come home and do anything else. My symptoms increased as the day progressed and got even worse in the evening.

Jon tried to help as much as he could when he was home, but most of the scheduling and household management still fell on me. At the time, I did not realize the additional strain that it added to my brain and how it affected my ongoing recovery.

Adding to the physical and emotional stress were the money concerns. My full-time salary and insurance benefits would not kick in for another month, and things remained tight.

Although we had been sending the bills and status reports to Henry regularly as requested, we had not received an update regarding the lawsuit. I called him and left a message for him to call me about the case. Ever since this whole fiasco, it seemed all I did was wait: wait for doctors; wait for test results; wait to see if I would screw up at work; wait for the news of the lawsuit. It was overwhelming at times. Henry did get back to me simply to say that it was progressing.

The first day of school for the students was only a few weeks away. As the deadline got closer, I found myself struggling to keep up the pace at work in preparation for the new school year. I had gotten back to full eight-hour days four times a week and felt the strain. I would wake up feeling refreshed, with fairly clear vision. Even with the Vyvanse, by mid-afternoon, my vision would become blurry, and my thinking would slow.

I started noticing that my memories of events that happened the previous year during our meetings were occasionally hazy and sometimes nonexistent. At one meeting, the principal asked me to pull up last year's one-to-one budget comparison we had worked on.

CHICKEN THERAPY

"When was that?"

"We did that last December on a Google spreadsheet," he said. "It should be in your files."

"Oh, right," I said, feeling a bit embarrassed. *I had no memory of this.* It was late in the afternoon. My brain felt fuzzy. I tried to search the files on my laptop, but the letters blurred.

"Let me check it out and send it to you tomorrow," I said, stalling for time. "I'm sure it will need some updating anyway." I had gotten good at covering my condition when needed.

"Okay," he said, a little surprised. "First thing." After a few minutes, the meeting broke up.

I returned to my classroom, closed my eyes, rested for a few minutes, then started pulling up my files. I was shocked when I found the folder marked BUDGET COMPARISON. Even though it looked a little familiar, I had no memory of creating it. In addition to coping with my vision issues, I now had to be aware of apparent memory issues as well when I got tired.

A sense of impending doom invaded my mind as I hurriedly walked out the door at the end of the school day. While squinting my eyes to avoid the bright sunlight, I massaged my neck with the other hand. It was the end of the day. My eyes were tired, and the bulging muscle in my neck was unwavering.

I knew that once the school year started, I'd need to start teaching classes as well, which meant 12-hour days. I was getting nervous about how I would manage it. In an attempt to find a solution, I made an appointment with Dr. Lori. After explaining my concerns, she increased the level of my ADD meds to help me cope with my memory and concentration issues. It seemed to help, but the new prescription also made me feel on edge and more argumentative than usual.

Thinking that my prism glasses might need adjustment as well, I called Dr. Brown. He squeezed me in for a quick appointment.

After explaining my concerns, he said he thought I might be regressing and prescribed a different level of prism sticker.

When I picked up my new glasses and put them on, I felt a whirling feeling inside my brain. Trying harder to focus, I realized that although I was not seeing double, I felt slightly disoriented "

How do they feel?" the optometrist asked.

"Not great. They're making me dizzy."

"It's a new prescription. It might take a little while to get used to them."

Before driving home, I took a short walk around the grounds. It was a nice day, and the sun felt good. Then, I sat in the car for a few more minutes, waiting for the weirdness to pass. My vision was better, but my brain still felt like it was swirling. I had to concentrate hard to orient myself. I closed my eyes and forced myself to calm down for a few more minutes.

Feeling a little better, I started to drive home. Even though I'd driven the route many times, I pulled over twice for a few minutes to get my bearings. The usual landmarks all looked different. It was frightening, and I almost called Jon to meet me. Instead, I persevered and finally got home.

The next morning, I had the same feeling of disorientation. I called Dr. Brown. He explained that my vision issues were still settling in. He suggested I switch between the old prism sticker and the new ones until I got more used to the prescription. That made sense, and it helped a little, especially at the end of the day.

The next school day, though, was a disaster. I was so anxious that my vision bounced between normal, blurry, and double. I felt nauseous most of the day and did my best to hide it from the staff and students. Somehow, I got through it. When I got home, I took off my glasses and immediately took a long nap. Later, I felt well enough to make dinner. Jon then cleaned up the dishes, and Jade tended to the flock when I announced that I was going upstairs to bed.

CHICKEN THERAPY

I continued to persevere. Every morning, I would use the first prism. By midday, when my eyes got tired, I would retreat to the bathroom and close my eyes for a few minutes. I would then switch to the new prism. The change would spur on a slight wave of nausea and momentary blurriness as my brain adjusted.

Sometimes I would be in front of the classroom, teaching from the board, walk to a student's desk to help, and realize that I couldn't see the paper clearly. My determination to make this work was waning, but I persisted.

Even though I woke up slightly refreshed and less anxious each morning, as the day progressed, my symptoms worsened, no matter which pair of prisms I wore. Despite my challenges, I remembered how much I missed the organized chaos and the energy my students brought with them into my classroom. It was good to feel needed and productive again, to be able to help others instead of being dependent on others to help me, so I continued to power through.

I eventually found myself unable to do much of anything outside of the school day except care for my flock in the morning, nap when I got home, and then prepare dinner. Jon would close up the coop at night.

A few weeks later, I woke up from a late Sunday afternoon nap with anxiety gnawing at the lining of my stomach. The monumental amount of work on my school schedule used to be enjoyable. Now it filled me with dread. *Would I be able to handle it? Would my symptoms get worse?*

I fight every day to find that part of me that no longer works,

I am breaking you too, piece by piece, each time the coaster jerks.

CHAPTER 14

My stress level was building as my workdays grew longer. The ADD medication, while it helped with my focus, contributed to my moodiness at the end of the day. Sometimes I would snap at Jon or Jade over some small issue. While they tried to be understanding, I knew I didn't make it any easier or more pleasant for any of us.

One example, in particular, sticks out in my mind. One Saturday morning, after a long, stressful week, I slept in, then enjoyed coffee on the deck with Jon. No headaches. My vision was manageable. We watched the chickens roam around the yard.

"Tonight, we're just going to relax," Jon announced. "Jade is at her friend's house, and you and I should have a nice dinner on the deck."

"That sounds wonderful!"

As Jon washed the cars and tended to the coop, I took an afternoon nap, followed by a luxurious bubble bath—something I seldom allowed for myself. I chose an outfit I knew Jon would like and spent some extra time on my hair and makeup. I looked at myself in the mirror. I felt great.

Later that evening, Jon and I chatted on the deck with a glass of wine while he cooked dinner on the grill. Our food was ready to eat just as the sun began to set—so romantic. I loved sitting there, looking out on our beautiful yard, surrounded by acres of trees.

It had been a while since we had dinner outside. I had forgotten how much I enjoyed the scenery and watching the chickens and ducks free-range in the grass. Occasionally, Ruby would hop on the deck, jump up on my lap, and try to steal my food. As I watched her scurry back to the coop with a choice scrap, everything suddenly seemed slightly blurry. Tilting my head, I realized that it was double when I looked straight on, not just to the left.

CHICKEN THERAPY

Damn. I had rested all day! I didn't *read or look at the computer. Why is this happening? Maybe it was the wine.*

"What's wrong?" Jon asked, seeing me tense up.

"My vision is bad, and I don't know why. I hate feeling like this!"

"We're home. Just ignore it. Have a little more wine."

"No, thanks. That's probably what's causing it."

He shrugged. "How was I supposed to know that?"

"I know I told you."

"If you knew it might be hard for you, why'd you drink it anyway?"

"You're supposed to help, not make it worse!"

The fun, relaxing evening we were enjoying quickly spiraled downward from there. He suddenly blew up and started ranting. He accused me of blaming him for everything and not appreciating all that he did for me.

"It's always about you."

The argument escalated. Maybe it was the first time he had shared his feelings about how my condition had affected our lives, and it shocked me. Maybe I was so on edge from the medications that I just couldn't control my anger and frustrations.

Furious, I stood up. "I don't need this." I just had to get away from him at that moment.

I walked over to the car and got in. I realized that I was seeing double and probably shouldn't be driving, so I just sat there, sobbing. *Was Jon right? Had I taken him for granted? Was I only concerned with my problems?*

By the time I got back, Jon had cleaned up and was watching TV. I walked right past him and went upstairs to bed. Later that night, in the quiet darkness, I heard him come in. We had agreed never to go to bed angry.

"You okay?" he whispered.

"I guess. You?"

"I don't know. I thought I could cope better. I'm sorry."

After a few long, lonely minutes, Jon lightly touched my leg. I felt the familiar connection and turned toward him. With no words to get in the way, I realized that at least there was one thing that could still be normal in my life.

I woke up a few hours later. As I glanced at Jon sleeping soundly, I vowed to try harder to be more understanding. None of this was his fault. *Would our lives ever get back to the way they had been before the accident?*

Unable to shake these thoughts and go back to sleep, I grabbed a coat and a flashlight and headed to the coop. The light of the full moon made the yard seem eerily peaceful. Most of the birds were happily asleep, all but Brie, my favorite Muscovy duck, who was sitting on a high roost in the run. Unlike most ducks, Muscovies like to roost in trees at night.

Needing to feel the comfort of his soft feathers, I hugged him tight. I could feel his heartbeat through his meaty chest that was covered in layers of down and waterproof feathers. His breath smelled rubbery and weirdly pleasant. At first, he angrily protested by flailing his strong wings and scratching me with the claws on his webbed feet, then he calmed down.

I understood his need to fight against being controlled. I knew how he felt. Yet, he was willing to let it go, accept it, and regain his peace. Maybe I had to learn to do that. Not fight so hard against the effects of my condition and learn to live with them. Feeling less anxious, I went back into the house, climbed into bed, and slept.

For a moment we linger at the top and both feel that alluring chill,

And then the coaster begins its decent down the unexpectedly steep hill.

CHAPTER 15

One night after work, all my challenges seemed to hit me at once. Jon was away on business. Jade was out at work. It had been a particularly stressful day at work and my double vision was bad.

It was getting dark when I left the school building. I had learned to drive by holding one hand over an eye when my double vision increased. Not an ideal workaround, especially in the early evening. If I went slow, I could manage. As I approached the house, I could hear Riley barking frantically. After opening the door, I watched him furiously race out to the yard, nose to the ground, and head toward the coop. Something was wrong. I dropped my school bags and ran after him. When I got there, my heart sank into my chest. It was empty and there were feathers strewn all over the yard. I could only assume some predator had been at work.

I called Jon hysterically. Jon calmly listened, then convinced me to hang up, get a flashlight, and search the grounds, then call back.

With a flashlight in hand, trying not to stumble because my vision was bad, I headed up the hill. Then, I heard the familiar clucking. I found most of the chickens sitting on a fence around the garden at the top of the hill and the ducks hiding in the bushes. After doing a head count, I realized that only Concussion Chicken and Queen Elizabeth were missing. It did not take me long to find their lifeless bodies in a pile of feathers a few yards away.

I don't know how I was able to do it. I got a cardboard box, placed their bodies inside, and put them in the barn to deal with later. Then, I went back up the hill to get the remaining chickens. I tried shooing them back into the coop, but they seemed too afraid to move. So, I grabbed each hen, one at a time, then walked it down, deposited it into the coop, and returned up the hill for the next one.

CHICKEN THERAPY

What seemed like hours later, I managed to get the last bird in the coop and then locked it. I went back into the house and called Jon. He did not answer. I left a message that we had lost two chickens, but the rest were safe.

Exhausted, with a pounding headache, I brought Riley inside, fed him and Daisy, had a few bites of something myself, and tried to relax by closing my eyes. When I opened them, things were still double and blurry. I sat in my chair and started sobbing.

As the tears streamed down my face, I realized that they were not only a reaction to losing my beloved chickens. The more I worked at dealing with my vision, it didn't seem to make a difference. I hated not being able to control my mood, my mind, and my eyes. I hated the person I had become. Frustrated at not being able to perform tasks that everyone else took for granted, I was lashing out more and more.

I knew I was on edge all the time. When Jon got home from a trip, there was always some kind of argument. I would rant on and on about how lonely and exhausted I was. He was getting tired of all my tantrums. As much as I wanted to tell him he was uncaring, I couldn't. He was right on some level that my anger and frustration just took over sometimes.

I was worried that I was relying more and more on my ADD medication to continue to handle my job, even though I knew it was contributing to my increasingly volatile emotional state. When I took a break from it, my ability to think quickly and focus lessened which made me even more irritable. When I got back on it, then it all started again. It was a vicious cycle I didn't know how to break.

When Jon got home the next day, I sat down and explained exactly how I was feeling.

He listened intently. "Maybe driving to and from work is making you too tired. Why don't you ask Eileen if you can catch a ride to and from work with her? That will take at least a little strain off your eyes."

Eileen was the school nurse and only lived a mile away from us. She was a kind and caring person, and I knew that would be no problem. It would also force me to limit my hours as she usually left on time.

"I can do that, I guess."

"Good. It also sounds like your glasses aren't working as well as they used to. Maybe you should see Dr. Brown."

Relieved to have someone else take charge, I tearfully agreed.

Eileen was only too happy to give me a ride. While it didn't help the strain on my eyes and overall fatigue, it was one less thing to worry about.

I called Dr. Brown and told him that I seemed to be regressing.

"It sounds like the prisms aren't working because your double vision has become unstable again."

"What should I do? I can't live like this."

"It's a complex condition. You should see Dr. Mike Monroe. He's a major specialist in your condition."

I sighed. *Another doctor.* "Is he local?"

"No, he works out of Johns Hopkins in Baltimore."

"That's at least an hour and a half away."

"Yes, but he's an expert in the field and should be able to help."

"Okay. I guess I have no choice."

Attending another appointment would mean both Jon and I would have to take a day off from work. When I informed the principal, he begrudgingly gave it to me, informing me that it would mean another deduction from my paycheck as I had no more sick days.

I had no idea what to think or how to feel on the way to the appointment. The drive was a little unnerving as we battled the rush-hour traffic on the freeway, then in Baltimore, to arrive in time for our 8:00 a.m. appointment. We had given ourselves plenty of time for the trip and finally arrived thirty minutes early at the massive hospital that seemed to encompass a few city blocks.

Cheerfully decorated skywalks above the street connected the buildings that were clearly labeled on the outside, making our search for the parking lot in the congested city less stressful. The modern, clean appearance made me feel hopeful somehow.

We went to what looked like the main building. I stopped when I saw the revolving door. Jon helped me navigate it. At the large reception desk, one of the several receptionists told us where to go.

When we got to Dr. Monroe's office, it was packed. His receptionist checked us in, handed me papers to fill out, and informed us that the doctor was running behind. Thankfully, there was coffee available.

After waiting nearly an hour, watching patient after patient enter and leave, it was finally my turn.

"I am going with you this time. No argument," Jon informed me.

A pre-exam was conducted by a very friendly, chatty young physician's assistant, who listened to my story and took notes.

"The doctor will be with you shortly."

Dr. Monroe introduced himself, shook my hand, and inquired about our trip. He was tall, with dark hair and kind eyes.

"It appears, from the pre-exam," he said, checking the chart, "that you not only have a right fourth cranial nerve palsy but also sixth cranial nerve palsy in both eyes as a result of the TBI."

"TBI?"

"Sorry, traumatic brain injury."

"I thought I had a concussion."

"Traumatic brain injury is an injury to the brain caused by trauma to the head. Yours was caused by the car accident. A mild brain injury may affect your brain cells temporarily. More serious traumatic brain injury can result in long-term or permanent complications."

"So, how does this apply to me?"

"Your cranial nerves were stretched by the force of the accident, causing your vision issues and related symptoms. The damage may be permanent. It's unclear at this point. It is also possible that the brain cells that are involved in sending signals from your eyes to your brain are also damaged. It's all part of the TBI."

"Prism glasses were helping initially. Why did they stop working?"

"Your degree of double vision fluctuates throughout the day. They only work if the degree stays stable. We'll need to do a few more tests to rule out any other underlying causes and to figure out the next steps. We still have a window of time for things to improve. You need to know that surgery may be an option."

"Surgery!" I was shocked.

"That will depend on the test results and if we can get your double vision to stop fluctuating. Remember, there is a possibility that this may never be resolved completely. In any event, whatever the course of treatment, it will take time and rest."

He looked at the chart again. "From what you told my assistant, your job creates too much stress on your vision. If you hope to recover from this, I strongly recommend that you stop working until we know more."

"I need to work!"

"Until we know more, you need to take time off. It could exacerbate the damage and interfere with the healing process."

My heart sank. The school year was in full swing. Teachers and students needed me to help them. How could I just take off and leave them hanging? Not to mention the salary.

"Let's get the additional tests done so we can see where we stand. Once we know more, I'll do everything I can to help resolve this."

CHICKEN THERAPY

I was numb.

"Thanks, doctor. We'll do whatever it takes to help."

"Good. I'll arrange for the tests and my office will get back to you. Best of luck."

"Thanks," I murmured as I mechanically got out of my seat and followed Jon out of the office.

"What am I going to do?" I said a few minutes into the drive home, nearly in tears. "More tests, more time off. This can't be real."

"We'll figure it out," Jon said reassuringly. "Maybe you can get some different kind of disability help and…"

"I don't want to go back on disability. I want to get back to normal," I snapped, then quickly regretted it. "Sorry, I didn't expect to hear that the damage may be permanent and involve my brain. It's so depressing."

"I know. One day at a time."

I didn't respond. I couldn't get the idea out of my head that these symptoms may never go away. When we got home, I pulled out my teaching contract and health insurance papers. Jon and I were surprised to see that my policy included long-term disability. I met all the requirements to acquire this benefit. I was entitled to twelve months of long-term disability once I gave notice to the school.

The check would be 60% of my salary. It would require mounds of paperwork and might take a few weeks, but it seemed pretty routine. There were two clauses in the policy that could be a problem. The clauses said that I could keep my school health insurance if I paid the entire premium without the usual school subsidy. It also stated that I must apply for Social Security Disability insurance to receive it.

"I think we could get by on that until I get well enough to get back to work." I tried to stay positive.

"We'll make it work. Your health is the most important thing."
I loved him for saying that.
"I'll call the school tomorrow."
The next day, Sally was quick to confirm the terms about long-term disability and said she'd get them in motion.
"What about the Social Security Disability Insurance part?"
"That part is up to you."
She gave me the website.
"You'll need to discuss the timing with the principal though. I'll let him know and he'll give you a call."
The next day, my principal called. We chatted for a bit, then he got down to business. "Although we can offer you long-term disability for one year, we cannot grant you another leave of absence."
The technology needs of the school are ongoing, and I need to hire a full-time replacement to ensure the students are receiving a consistent, high-quality program.
"You mean you're letting me go?" I stammered in disbelief.
"I'm afraid so. We'll be sorry to lose you. You helped build a solid program here."
"What about the program in the interim? My classes. I could stay until…"
"The tech team can fill in until we find someone. I've reassigned your classes also. I am sorry. I can let the faculty know, or maybe you want to write them a letter?"
"Yes, I can do that," I said, keeping my professional demeanor while dying a little on the inside. "I hope I can rely on getting a letter of recommendation from you for the future."
"Of course. Best of luck."
Hanging up the phone, I broke down. I had built a good, fulfilling career for years, only to see it collapse.
When Jon got home and heard the news, he was mad.

"After all you've done for them and all of the hours you worked above and beyond what was required those first few years?"

"I know, but there's nothing I can do."

I wrote the letter to my colleagues. Phone calls and emails came in from both parents and teachers wishing me well. For the next few weeks, it seemed that anywhere I went, I would run into a friend or acquaintance who would inquire how I was or why I wasn't at school. After hearing my brief explanation, they all conveyed how sorry they were and asked if there was anything they could do for me. I was overwhelmed with their good wishes and concerns. At the same time, I was embarrassed and angry.

As always, I found some solace in being around my flock. Even though we let our chickens roam freely only during the day, I knew that there was always the danger of predators. The only way to protect them completely would be to keep them locked in the coop all the time. That would mean no sunlight, fresh air, no dust baths, and no foraging for bugs. While *we* might be content that they were safe, their lives would be limited and without freedom.

I thought about my own life after the accident and my journey back to work and socializing, only to be pulled back by my ongoing vision problems into worrying about my health and future. I got locked up in my own coop out of fear. Would I ever get to free-range fully again without fear of having to live with my health problems forever? I had to remain hopeful and, despite the challenges, do whatever it took to break out of my limited environment.

****

Dr. Lori sympathetically listened to me as I relayed the new developments at my next checkup. When I explained my thoughts on the ADD medicine, she offered to write me a prescription for the same medicine but at a lower dose.

CHICKEN THERAPY

"Now that you aren't working and juggling all that stress, I think that just may help you to focus and manage your moods."

It made sense. I left Dr. Lori's office feeling a little less heavy-hearted.

Upon hearing the news of my job loss, Adrianna insisted on coming home for a long weekend. Jade took a day off from school to spend time with us. Our relationship had grown and changed over the years. We all had different personalities and perspectives on life, and constantly argued about them, but always had each other's backs.

As we sat down at the kitchen table waiting for Jon to finish grilling dinner, the girls reminisced about the many adventures they had growing up. As I listened to their conversation, I felt a happiness in my heart that I had not felt for a long time. They talked about playing in the woods, enjoying campfires in the yard, and sneaking chickens into the house. I yearned to stay in this moment forever. Jon came in with the food and sat down.

The conversation then turned to me. I filled Adrianna in on what's been happening.

"I wish I could just turn one eye off. That would solve everything."

"What about an eye patch?" Adrianna asked.

"I tried that and it was very uncomfortable. Although things weren't double, it was tiring and still hard to see."

"I have an idea," Jon said. "What if you wore your contacts with a clear pair of glasses, no prescription, and we blacked out one lens? It would be more comfortable than a patch and still have the same results."

"I will try anything at this point."

"I have quite a few pairs of safety glasses, and they even have readers in them. They're not stylish."

"Okay. It might work."

"I will go find a pair right now."

"This should be good!" Adrianna chuckled. "Daddy never disappoints!"

He was back in a few minutes.

"Do you have your contacts in?"

I nodded.

Jon handed me a sleek pair of safety glasses. He had expertly blackened out one lens with a permanent marker. I put them on.

"How do I look?" I asked.

"Ridiculous!" Adrianna blurted out.

"Adrianna!" Jade scolded her.

"How do you see?" Jon asked.

"Well…" I said as I looked around. "Nothing's double. It's weird not being able to see all around me. I will try this. It can't hurt!"

"Honestly Mom, they don't look that bad. We can get nice ones if you want," Adrianna said.

I wore them for the next few hours but was thankful to take them off when it was time to go to bed.

The next morning the girls and I decided that shopping was in order. It was a beautiful clear seventy-degree fall day. A perfect day to be out and about. Both girls tried to hold back their giggles as I proceeded to put on the glasses with one eye blackened out.

"I'll drive," Adrianna announced.

When we got to the mall, we stopped at a hip clothing shop. I tripped slightly and bumped into things in the aisles. The glasses affected my peripheral vision more than I noticed at home. People stared at me while Jade helped me.

"It's okay, Mom. They make these damn displays too close together," she said.

"You got that right," some other woman said. "Happens to me all the time."

CHICKEN THERAPY

After a few minutes, we left the store.

Once outside, we all burst out in laughter. It felt so good to laugh instead of always feeling exhausted, guilty, or ashamed. I realized that I didn't need to pretend when I was with them, that I could be myself, and be comfortable.

"Let's go to DSW. I need new shoes for work," Adrianna suggested.

"Yeah, I can sit down and wait," I added. More laughs.

We happily helped Adrianna pick out shoes. The girls' camaraderie gave me confidence. As the morning progressed, my eyes and head began to ache.

"I think I need a break from these," I announced as I took my glasses off.

The familiar whirling inside my head, blurriness, and nausea ensued as we continued to shop. I tried to ignore my symptoms.

When we stopped at the food court for a snack, I couldn't cope with all the noise and food smells.

"Maybe we should head home."

"No problem. Let's get a Coke for the road." On the ride home, I didn't put the glasses back on and sat with my eyes closed. I pondered how lucky I was, despite my vision problems. My family was my rock, and I needed to be grateful for them. Sadly, I had to abandon Jon's glasses.

That Sunday, Adrianna asked me if I could show her where all our financial documents and bills were located.

"Why?"

"Well, Dad has many talents. Organizing and bill paying is not one of them. Since you're still healing, I thought I could help streamline the process to make your life easier. It's what I do."

A little hesitant about admitting I might need help with the routine tasks, I had to admit it was getting to be a challenge doing all the bookkeeping because my eyes got tired so quickly.

CHICKEN THERAPY

First, Adrianna had me write down all of the passwords to accounts that were used to pay the bills. Then, she helped me arrange important documents into color-coded file folders with large letter labels.

"Now think of any important recurring things you want to put in your calendar. I will put them in for you and set up reminders on your computer."

As I listened to her, I heard echoes of me. Practical. Organized. Proactive. I was proud to have sown the seeds that had contributed to the grown adult woman she'd become. We had a nice and productive time together, and I thanked her for her help.

On Monday morning, Jon left for work, followed by Jade, who went to class. Adrianna packed her things and loaded them into the car. "See you soon," she said as we hugged goodbye.

Spending this long weekend with her, I realized just how much I missed her.

As soon as Adrianna pulled out of the driveway, I realized that everyone had a place to go, a busy life to live—except me. *Get a grip. Think positive. You had such a good weekend with the girls.* Forcing myself to pull out of my declining mood, I put on my coat, went out the door, and headed toward the towering oak tree that the girls had named Tom years ago.

I sat against the trunk and looked up into the huge umbrella Tom's branches created. It reminded me of the day when the girls were young, and we stood under that same tree during a surprise rainstorm. I could almost hear the laughter we shared while standing drenched under Tom's branches.

I longed for those times. I longed to be normal, to drive more, to go to work, to make plans, to see without a problem, to laugh again. A gust of wind moved through the branches, causing some of the crimson and brown leaves to cascade to the ground. A few weeks ago, the leaves were green. Now, they were making their way to the ground, dried up and dead. Just like pieces of my life.

Ugh. What a dark thought. Focus on the good stuff. Focus on hope for the future.

Try as I might,

I can't stop lashing out,

The car picks up steam,

And I can only hear my terrified screams and shouts.

CHAPTER 16

It felt unsettling to have no routine. For the first time in my life, I had no structured schedule or goals to work toward. Without work distractions, I awoke most days without feeling any motivation. *What was the point of even getting out of bed? What did I have to look forward to? More double vision and headaches?*

Sure, I had my chickens and the household chores, but I didn't have anything to challenge me. Taking care of bills added to my depression. We just didn't have enough coming in, forcing me to juggle payments.

Wondering about the status of our legal case, I decided to call Henry. I was surprised he picked up the phone on the second ring.

"Hello, Mrs. Helm. How are you feeling?"

"Not great. My condition has gotten worse, and I lost my job."

"I'm sorry to hear it. When did you stop working?"

"A few weeks ago. I am now on long-term disability. Our finances are tight. I'm waiting for the payments to begin. The medical bills are piling up as you know from the copies I send you. What's going on with the case?"

"Well, your job loss is a new development which we should add to the damages. Send me the termination documents and other eligible expenses. I'll put all the bills together and send them to our economist."

"Why an economist?"

"The economist helps figure out the amount we should sue for. He will determine the exact number of wages you have lost to this point and then calculate the amount of future earnings you will lose. Then we will figure in the expenses as well as your pain and suffering."

"Then what?"

"Well, once we determine the value of the suit, I send all the documentation to the defense attorneys with the amount we want, and then the case is remanded to the court to set a date. The insurance company will try to delay. They will most likely want to take depositions from you, your husband, the driver, and the police."

"Wow."

"Then you'll need to see doctors selected by the insurance company to determine the nature and full extent of your injuries. At any point in the process, we may receive a settlement offer to avoid going to a jury trial, but that's not certain. I'd say it could take another year or so to resolve it."

"Another year!" I said, shocked. "I'm not sure we can survive that long."

"I know this is a hardship. As I said when we first met, the insurance companies stretch it out as long as possible. Have you considered applying for supplemental income from Social Security?"

"Do you mean the Social Security Disability Insurance?"

"Yes, that's it."

"I've already applied for it. In the meantime, please do what you can to expedite the case."

"I'll be in touch when I know more."

During dinner, I told Jon about my phone conversation with Henry.

"He said it could take a year."

"Lawyers and the legal system. It's a mess," he said. "We'll survive and if you get better...."

"What do you mean 'if'!" I said, feeling my temper rise. "Don't you think I'll get over this?"

"Of course I do. I'm just trying to be practical. We're in this together."

CHICKEN THERAPY

"It doesn't sound like it," I shot back.

"You are being ridiculous." He walked out of the room.

I just stood there, fuming and hurt.

I knew Jon was trying to help, but I couldn't take it. The pressure of my symptoms, my job loss, and the lawsuit were all so stressful. *How do people with more serious injuries or fewer financial resources survive it?*

I threw on a jacket and marched up to the chicken coop, the only place I felt like I belonged anymore. After grabbing some dried mealworm treats, I plopped down on the grass. The chickens and ducks promptly converged around me, anticipating their bedtime snack. Tossing the worms into the crowd, I thought about my conversation with Henry. After all the problems and delays, who knew if we'd ever get the compensation I deserved?

Ruby and Brie were impatiently prodding me for more treats, so I grabbed another handful from the small bag I carried and held my hand out. They were the only ones who liked to eat them from my hand. The others kept a safe distance from my reach.

Lady Gaga suddenly ran up and stole the entire bag of worms. She was a small-breed chicken who earned her name because of her glamorous shock of long head feathers, called a crest, that stood straight up on the top of her head and then cascaded over her eyes. Satiny cream-colored feathers covered her thin body like a beautiful long cashmere coat. She then strategically raced back to the coop, weaving between any chickens in her way.

The rest of the flock pursued her with a single-minded focus on that bag. Brie snatched it from her, and chaos reigned until I ran over and retrieved the bag. Treat time over, I shooed them into the coop for the night.

I thought about what just happened. Both Lady Gaga and Brie knew what they wanted and went after it. *Maybe I need to figure out how to go after my bag of worms.*

You react by fueling the fire,

Which pushes the car downhill even faster,

At the bottom we reconnect,

And fight like hell to find the "us" before the next disaster.

CHAPTER 17

At the suggestion of my daughters, I immersed myself in motivational audiobooks and podcasts. I had never been someone who engaged in self-help activities, but I had to admit, they did help my anxiety and mood swings and gave me some control and perspective.

One evening after securing the coop, I decided to go back in, sit on a bucket, and think. While the bucket was cold and the air slightly pungent, the atmosphere was peaceful and calm. This coop offered the flock the security and refuge I so desperately sought. I wished I could live in their simple world.

In my world, my job, my career, defined me. It made me feel secure in my abilities, part of a community, independent, and needed. I had always been one to provide support for my family and students. Now, I needed it from others. The realization was hard to deal with.

Tomorrow, the flock will wake up with the sun to Kevin's crowing. They will hurriedly run to the gate to escape their refuge, free-range, and just enjoy their life. It all seemed so uncomplicated. Each day was the same as the next for them.

I had thrived on challenges, adapting to and solving problems as they came about. This was different, my ongoing vision issues had me stymied. I had always thought that planning and hard work could fix anything. Now, I wasn't so sure. Unlike the chickens, I just couldn't resign myself to my situation. I had to find a way to take back control.

***

As the days passed, I realized that my vision was becoming blurrier, and the double vision persisted. I was beginning to wonder if there was something else seriously wrong with me. Maybe I had an undiagnosed brain tumor. I googled it and found that headaches and blurry sight often were early symptoms. My anxiety and fear that there was an underlying problem grew, even though none of my many doctors had even suggested anything of the sort.

Often at night, I got down on my knees next to the bed and prayed like I had as a child. I prayed to God I didn't have any other serious problems. I prayed for strength and understanding in managing my condition.

After praying, I woke up more relaxed, more ready to meet the day. It was almost as though my prayers helped lift a weight from my shoulders.

***

"How are you feeling?" Jon asked on the drive to my appointment with Dr. Monroe.

"Hopeful," I said calmly.

Dr. Monroe informed me that the CT scan and bloodwork were fine. There were no complicated physical issues.

Thank you, God.

"However, your double vision continues to be too unstable to prescribe surgery. Surgery could make things worse at this point."

"Is there anything else we can do?"

"We could try another set of prisms. It may be the most complicated prism prescription I have ever written, as I am going to try to address multiple issues. I think it is worth a try."

"Okay. If you think it will help."

When I got the new prisms, I closed my eyes, held my breath, and then put them on. I slowly opened my eyes and looked around the room. Although I did not see double, everything appeared distorted. I had to keep adjusting the position of the glasses. The optometrist assured me I'd get used to them in time.

CHICKEN THERAPY

For the next few days, I kept trying to adjust my glasses, thinking if I tilted the lenses at the right angle, I would see more comfortably. Nothing helped. I went back to the optometrist three times to get them adjusted. Each visit brought some momentary relief. Each time, once I was home, the symptoms would start all over again.

I tried to be patient and allow my eyes and mind to get used to the new prism prescription. I noticed that when I was looking at something familiar like my sofa, or the coop, it wasn't too bad. If I left the familiar surroundings of my home, things quickly became either blurry or double. If I powered through it, I eventually felt tired, dizzy, and nauseous and had to take the glasses off to rest.

As the weeks slid by, the world became smaller. I was now afraid that it was unsafe for me to drive and completely stopped. Adrianna's bill-paying system was a great help as using the computer for more than a few minutes was now very difficult.

Only my daily long walks around the sanctuary of my yard gave me some relief. I could wander around my familiar surroundings without having to focus on anything. I knew it wasn't reality, but it helped me cope.

Many of the self-help audiobooks suggested that journaling was a great way to stay focused on healing. I remembered how, as a teenager, I used to write about my feelings in a diary. I had always loved to write, so I decided to give it a try.

I started with a stylus and tablet. Depending on what else I had done that day, writing for more than a few minutes strained my eyes and took away any energy to continue. I decided to try the talk-to-text function.

My excitement for a solution dissipated when I realized that every time the wind blew, or Riley barked, or a truck passed by, it recorded a wrong word. I cursed out of frustration and my tablet recorded that also. When I realized that I spent more time fixing the mistakes than actually writing, I gave up on this hi-tech solution. I tried typing on my computer, but the words didn't flow that easily and my eyes got tired too quickly. Finally, I resorted to pencil and paper. I found I couldn't focus on the words as I wrote them. I decided to put it on the back burner for now.

My vision seemed to continue to deteriorate, and my other symptoms got worse. I was losing hope of ever getting better. Jon and I were fighting constantly. His frequent out-of-town trips just made it all worse. I had no escape from the double vision and all the issues that accompanied it. My eyes had become a jail and depression, my jailer.

I felt as though I may be on the edge of insanity and desperately wanted to know how to not fall in. Overwhelmed, unable to bear the pain any longer, I retreated to my bed and sobbed uncontrollably.

Waves of emotion pounded my body as I realized that the only self I had ever known was gone. There had been no retirement party, no funeral, no cards. I realized that I was mourning myself.

That night, Jade found me in bed when she got home.

"Mom, what's wrong?"

"Everything. It's just so hard. I can't do anything. I can't take it."

"You need to get out. It's nearly dinner time. Let's go to that Chinese place we like."

I nodded, got dressed, and followed her out to the car. *Only a few years ago she was a child I comforted, now I had become the child needing her comforting advice.*

Thankfully, the Chinese restaurant wasn't crowded. I remembered sitting at this same table with her when life was normal. We had stopped there after shopping for a dress for a big date. She was excited and we laughed a lot.

I took off my glasses and tried not to focus on anything except my food or Jade. My eyes eventually wandered to the décor, to the other customers. I started to get dizzy and nauseous. I had to close my eyes.

"Are you okay, Mom?"

I opened my eyes. "Just a little queasy. It'll pass."

"I've been thinking. Weed may help you. It helps lots of people with nausea, dizziness, and anxiety."

I hadn't thought about pot in quite a long time. I smoked a little in college for the sole purpose of having fun. I had read that its medical benefits were becoming more widely known. Some states were legalizing it for medicinal purposes, but not in Pennsylvania, yet.

"It's illegal, hon."

"Technically, yeah. But it's all over. I'm sure I can get you some."

"Thanks. It's too risky."

She thought for a second. "I know for a fact that Cousin Brad smokes a lot. He's got a safe connection."

I was shocked. Brad was a second cousin who was happily married with a child on the way. He had a successful career as an electrical engineer.

"I don't know. I wouldn't want it to get back to anyone in the family."

"Don't worry. He wouldn't either. I'll give him a call and say it's for a friend."

"Well, maybe. Let me talk to your dad first."

"Okay. I'm sure he'll be fine with it."

That night, I told Jon when he came home from his trip about Jade's suggestion. He said he had no problem with me using it if it helped. I told Jade the next day. A few days later, Brad showed up with the goods. I was surprised it was so expensive.

"Hope it helps your friend," he said taking the cash.

"Me too."

Brad educated me on how to use it. Being a nonsmoker, it took some time to get used to inhaling and holding the smoke. Eventually, I got the hang of it. While it didn't help my vision, it quelled the nausea and relieved some of my anxiety for the moment.

I used it sparingly, only when I needed a reprieve from the spasming muscles around my eyes, or when I felt unable to deal with my frustration. It seemed to make my life a little more tolerable.

Then it all came crashing down.

Normally, we would host Thanksgiving and our house would be bursting with friends and relatives. I felt sad and embarrassed having to tell my usual guests that I would not be hosting this year. While they all understood, it was yet another sign that my life had changed for the worse.

Adrianna suggested that just Jon, Jade, and I travel to her small apartment for the holiday. Her boyfriend would be with his family. She said she would prepare the meal, and I could just sit back and enjoy the holiday for a change. I was deeply grateful for her caring and concern.

"May we should invite your Dad's family? It's only three more."

"Mom, I don't think there's room for everyone."

"Even though it'll be tight, at least we'll be together. I'll bring the corn and potatoes."

"Okay, if you say so."

The morning before Thanksgiving Day, I awoke in an irritable mood. I hadn't slept well, and my neck hurt. My double vision was bad that day, and I was feeling nauseous. The thought of dealing with that many people in Adrianna's tiny apartment for the entire day with no reprieve caused me to panic. *What was I thinking?*

I decided to make the best of it. I'd feel better tomorrow. I took a few puffs of a joint, tried to calm down, and then went back to bed for a few hours.

Feeling refreshed, I showered and then began making the sides. I put the corn in the oven to bake and started peeling the potatoes. The potatoes looked blurry in my hand, but I continued peeling until my hand slipped and I cut myself. I had peeled potatoes for years and never cut myself. I had a hard time finding a bandage in the bathroom and seeing clearly enough to put it on the cut.

Feeling as though I would explode from frustration, I stopped. Even this simple task seemed too difficult for me. I turned off the oven and left the potatoes on the counter.

When Jon came home, he found me on the sofa, staring at the floor.

"What's wrong?"

"I can't do it."

"Can't do what?"

"Make the corn and potatoes. Deal with so many people all day tomorrow."

"What do you mean? It was your idea."

"I know, but it's too much for me. Please call Adrianna and ask her to uninvite your family."

"Chris, it's the day before the holiday. She can't just…"

"Please… or I can't go."

"If you need to do this, you make the call."

He was right. I had to make the call. Adrianna was angry.

"I can't just uninvite Dad's family the day before. It's rude. And I've got all this food."

"I know. I'm sorry. I'm not feeling up to it all. Maybe I'll just stay home."

"No, Mom. It's all planned. You need to come."

"Spending the day with so many people at your place will be too painful for me."

"Mom, you're exaggerating."

I lost it and started yelling. "I am not! You don't know how I feel!"

She hung up.

"Well?" Jon asked.

I didn't respond and pushed past him and out the door, angry, embarrassed, and depressed. *How could I do this to my daughter, who was only trying to help?* I had become a stranger to myself. I couldn't shake the notion that I may never return to normal, that this was all there was: sadness, frustration, anger.

Thoughts of not wanting to live invaded my brain. I headed toward the woods, trying to lose myself in the natural surroundings. As I walked, tiny drops of icy rain pelted my face. Seeking refuge under a tree, I sat down on a log, wondering how I had gotten lost in this horrible new world, and if I could ever find my way back.

Cold and wet, I returned to the house after a short time. Jon was standing out front.

"What is wrong with you? You could get sick."

Unable to answer his accusatory remarks, I silently walked past him and sat in the darkened living room.

Jon followed me in and handed me a towel.

"Well? What's going on?"

"I don't know."

"What about tomorrow?"

"Do what you want."

With total disregard for his presence or his feelings, I climbed up the steps to our bedroom, took off my wet clothes, and collapsed into bed.

I awoke after midnight. Jon was asleep. The events of that afternoon came flooding back in hazy bits and pieces. My hand hurt. My argument with Adrianna. My disregard for Jon. I was devastated that I had acted that way. It all felt like a bad dream.

I got up and went into the living room and tried to call Adrianna. I left a message, apologizing and said I'd be coming after all. I then went back to bed and set the alarm for the next morning.

The alarm went off around seven, and I woke Jon up.

"What's happening?"

"We need to get ready to go. I left a message for Adrianna that we will be coming after all."

"My sister called last night after Adrianna called her to tell them it was off. She made up some excuse about her having a stomach virus."

"We can still go."

"Are you sure?"

"Yes. We can pick up something to take on the way."

A few hours later, after Jade fed the flock, we quickly packed the car, grabbed Riley, and began the long drive to Adrianna's apartment. On the way, we picked up a pumpkin pie from a local farmstand.

Halfway there, Adrianna finally called back.

"We're on her way," I said cheerily.

"Don't bother. I tossed the turkey and the rest of the food last night after calling Aunt Gladys. I'm on the way with Phil to have Thanksgiving with his family."

"But…"

"I can't deal with this right now. You need to get help, Mom. Don't call me for a while." She hung up.

My mind reeled and my heart shattered. She had been so excited about hosting her first Thanksgiving, and I had turned what should have been a happy memory into an unforgivable tragedy.

"What did she say?" Jade asked.

"Adrianna threw out all her food and is going to Phil's family."

We all sat in deafening silence.

"Let's just go to a restaurant," I suggested.

"They are probably all full," Jon replied. "Besides, you can't take the crowds, remember?"

That hurt, but I couldn't blame him for saying that.

Why couldn't I have just sucked it up and gone to Adrianna's?

We found some greasy spoon on the way back, got their packaged Thanksgiving dinner to go, and went home.

After the dismal, prefab dinner, and the pumpkin pie, Jon and Jade went to the living room and watched some old movie while I cleaned up. At least I could still do that, I thought. My chest tightened and my heart ached as I wondered if Adrianna would forgive me.

My knees felt weak, so I sat down at the table and reminisced in my thoughts. Holidays were always filled with joy and family. I loved having large family gatherings at our house. My favorite holiday to host was Christmas Eve. Every Christmas Eve, the house was adorned in quaint Christmas attire. The kitchen counters brimmed over with special holiday foods and freshly baked cookies.

The evening always ended with the traditional picture in front of the tree. Jade and Adrianna would sneak up to the coop minutes before, to snag a sleeping chicken, bring it into the house, and include it in the picture. I was terrified those days were over and longed to go back in time. Another casualty of my damn condition.

The next morning, I awoke feeling slightly motivated. I decided to try to go back to journaling. Despite my years of working digitally, I always enjoyed the feeling of writing using a pencil on paper. It was so satisfying somehow, and I thought I'd try it again.

Unable to find a pencil sharpener but wanting to write, I grabbed a crayon from the back of the junk drawer. I immediately found that writing with crayons made the words flow easier, and the thick lines didn't strain my eyes as much as the thin pencil lines. The only problem was that I could not fit many words on a piece of regular paper because the crayon forced me to write using larger letters. Feeling inspired, I called Jon and asked him to stop at a store on the way home and pick up a large artist pad and a box of crayons.

That evening, after Jon handed me the large, sturdy pad with a hard back cover, I opened the cover and ran my hand over the fresh, clean pages. It felt right. I closed the cover and wrote "JOURNAL" on the front in large, bold letters. As I placed it on the desk, I felt a familiar sensation in the pit of my stomach. *Could it be that spark I felt so long ago?*

***

One agonizing week later, Adrianna called. I profusely apologized again and let her know that I never intended to hurt her.

"Is it that bad, Mom?"

"It can be. I can't control how it makes me feel sometimes."

I realized that I hadn't shared the emotional rollercoaster I was on with her as I had with Jade and Jon. We chatted for a while, and she promised to come home soon. I was so happy and relieved that we'd reconciled.

One morning, a few days later, while in the shower, I started moving my eyes left and right, up and down, hoping to relieve the aching muscles around them. It occurred to me that it had been a while since I had moved my eyes around this much.

Maybe I am not moving my eyes around as much as I should. Maybe it was like exercising and stretching. Maybe I needed to rely on the prisms less and use my eye muscles more.

I decided to ditch the prism glasses until my next visit to Dr. Monroe. I went back to contacts and tried to move my eyes around more to see if there was any change. At first, I continued to avoid looking to the left, where the double vision was most prominent. When I got tired, I sat down and closed my eyes for ten minutes. After only a day, I could see a difference. While my double vision persisted, the odd whirling sensations in my brain and the nagging muscle pain around my eyes had markedly decreased.

After a few weeks, my new routine seemed to be working. I improved enough to increase my reading and computer use to maybe 10-15 minutes at a time. I could visit stores and shops for short periods without bumping into things or feeling disoriented. I slowly started driving again. Baby steps. I was happy with any improvement at this point.

Late one afternoon, on my way out to the coop to bring the chickens in from free-range, I heard the sound of a terrified squawk. The entire flock raced up the hill frantic and frightened.

I looked around and didn't see any predators. I ran up the hill and did a head count when I got to them. All were there except Orloff, who was a beautiful Russian breed that looked more like a mythical creature than a chicken. She was taller than most chickens and sported beautiful brown, black, and white feathers. The long feathers on her head splayed away from her face, traveled around and below her eyes, and down the back of her head like hair.

Scanning the wooded knoll below, I spotted what looked like her body lying at the bottom of the hill. It was blurry. Careful not to stumble, I ran down the hill to her.

Her eyes were closed. She was breathing but couldn't stand up. I noticed that her right leg seemed injured. Some hawk must have attacked her and hadn't finished the job. I gingerly lifted her and brought her to the porch. After a few minutes, she opened her eyes but remained motionless. When I placed her in a standing position on the ground, she just slowly crumpled to the ground.

CHICKEN THERAPY

Orloff sat there, dazed and quiet. I brought her water and sat next to her. Seeing she was okay, I ran out to shoo the other chickens back into the coop for safety.

The porch became her home for the next few weeks. For a few hours every day, I would let her perch on a deck chair where she would sit and look at the wall for hours. Orloff eventually recovered enough to join the rest of the flock. Her leg never healed completely, so she sort of leaned to the left when she walked around. When the other chickens bothered her, as they often do with injured birds, she just ignored them.

I admired her ability to adapt to her circumstances. Her instinct to thrive was inspiring. At that moment, I felt a lot like her. I had found a way to make the best of my situation with my new routine.

Somehow along the way we stay connected,

and hold on tight,

Please God let the ride be over,

before we lose this fight.

CHAPTER 18

One evening after one of my better days, Jon and I decided to visit the local tavern that was owned by Tom, one of his childhood friends. It was a cozy, inviting little place that played just the right country music. It had been ages since we had been there.

It was a Tuesday night, so it wasn't too crowded. As soon as we walked in, Tom happily greeted us.

"Where have you guys been hiding? I haven't seen you around town for a long time!"

As Tom and Jon talked, I sat at the bar, waiting for a table to open up. The music was not too loud, and I enjoyed just being in a familiar and lively place.

"Hey, Chris!" I heard a voice call out.

Tilting my head, I tried to see who it was; I struggled to recognize the blurry face. I waved anyway, and the woman came over.

"Hi… Beverly, Sara's mom. From the pool. Remember me?"

"Hi, sure I do. How've you been? Sara must be in high school by now."

We chatted for a while. It was nice to catch up with someone who didn't know about my accident.

Jon came over, and the waitress led us to a table. I used my readers to order from the menu. It felt like being together on a date like we used to do. We had a pleasant meal, and I even got up to do a slow dance with him on the floor. I felt a little dizzy but recovered quickly.

After dinner, on our way out, a young man walked up to us.

"Mrs. Helm?"

"Yes."

"It's Jim Strathen."

I looked up and smiled. He was a bit blurry too. I recognized him as one of my former students, now a grown young man.

"Hi, Jim. How are you?"

"Fine. Just graduated from college in computer science. You know that you were always my favorite math teacher."

"Thanks. That's great." We spoke for a few minutes, then I wished him luck and left.

On the way home in the truck, I told Jon how much fun I had and that we should get out more.

"I agree."

"Seeing Beverly and Jim helped me remember how much I have done with my life and how many people I've helped. Between teaching and coaching, I had made a lot of good relationships."

"I'm glad you had a good time."

Once home, feeling celebratory about having an unusually good, almost normal evening, we decided to have a nightcap of sparkling cider.

"I wish that none of this happened," I said.

"I'll drink to that." We clinked our glasses.

"Even though it was a good day, I still saw double in the bar."

"I guess the sooner you learn to accept it all, the better it will be."

"What does that mean?"

"It's just… forget it."

"No. You need to explain."

"What's the point? I can't talk to you when you're like this."

"Like what?"

"Irrational." He stood and started to walk toward the study door.

"Don't you dare walk away from me."

I got up and stood in his way.

"MOVE!" he shouted.

"Not until you tell me what you meant." I didn't budge.

Jon grabbed my arm and shoved me out of the way. It was the first time he ever did anything like that. He went into the study and slammed the door.

I stood there horrified. What had happened? All I wanted was for Jon to clarify what he said about my struggles to deal with my vision issues. I knew he loved me. Why had I blown up after such a nice evening? Maybe he touched a nerve about the hopelessness I felt every day. The fear that I would never get better. Was I so wrapped up in my own problem that I couldn't see how much he always supported me?

That night was the first night we had ever slept separately at home in our married life. I barely got any sleep. The next morning, I stayed in bed until Jon left, too embarrassed to confront him.

I put on a comfy old sweatshirt, brewed some coffee, and enjoyed a cup glancing out the window. It had snowed a few inches overnight. I bundled up and headed to the coop to greet the day. As I approached it, I noticed the spectacular way the sun lit up the icicles hanging from the roof.

I wondered what the chickens and ducks thought when they saw their outside world had transformed into a winter wonderland overnight. Did they even notice? I chuckled to myself, during a momentary reprieve from my bleak thoughts.

Jon had cleared a path for them before he left. The chickens cautiously peered out as I opened the door, squinting their eyes from the brightness of the sun as it reflected off the newly fallen snow. Kevin dared to go out first, followed by the rest of the flock. The moment each chicken touched the cold snow, they squawked hysterically, then ran, flapping their wings to find snowless ground.

Lady Gaga was barely visible as her feathers were the same color as the snow. Her feet had sunk below the surface, and she was patiently standing there, slowly sinking, letting out an occasional squawk. Her long shock of head feathers stuck up completely straight. She didn't struggle or try desperately to get out. Somehow, she just waited until she could get out.

As I gently lifted her out to run around with the others, I thought about my condition. Perhaps it was time for me to resign myself to my fate too. No one was waiting to pluck me out of my distress. Doctors, family, therapists. Maybe it was up to me to accept it and move on. Jon's words echoed in my thoughts.

Thoughtful, I trudged back towards the house. The trees were decorated with white glistening snow beneath a bright clear blue sky. I could still see traces of grey and white storm clouds and I hoped that the anger and hurt that Jon and I had felt just a few hours earlier could dissipate like the clouds.

This new sea, it takes me to new places,

Streams and rivers I never knew,

Only when I had no choice but to succumb to nature,

Did my life become alive, and finally my soul did too.

CHAPTER 19

It had been over a year since the accident. My long-term disability insurance checks from school were steady but not nearly enough. My ever going back to work seemed more of a dream than a reality at this point.

Jon found a new job fixing industrial machinery locally with good benefits. It didn't involve travel or pay quite as much. Two steps forward and one step back.

I had filed the paperwork for additional disability from social security months before and I was waiting to hear about the next step: being evaluated by their doctors. It took forever, but I received notice about the scheduled doctor visits. I was very surprised to see that I was signed up for a visit to a psychologist, not a neuro-ophthalmologist. It didn't make any sense. My condition was physical, not psychological. I called the office to clarify what I was sure was a mistake. After nearly half an hour on hold, I finally got a human being.

"Name. Social Security number," she asked curtly.

I gave her the information.

"What is your issue?"

I explained my concern about the appointment with a psychologist.

"That is the requirement for your claim. Concussion, right?"

"Yes, but--"

"Memory issues?"

"Not really but my…"

"If you want the benefit, you need to keep the appointment," she said and hung up.

Yet another indignity from a system that is supposed to help people, not make them feel worse.

CHICKEN THERAPY

The next few weeks involved getting people to drive me to the various appointments with the social security doctors. Most of the visits were routine and involved the usual amount of paperwork. Although it was tedious, it was nothing I hadn't experienced before. Until my last appointment with the psychologist.

Jade drove me. We pulled into the parking lot of a dreary old government building in the next town. I was grumpy.

"I don't understand why I have to see a psychologist."

"It's all part of the government bureaucracy. It's the last one, right? Don't worry, Mom. You got this."

"I guess," I said as I exited the car.

Once inside the door, there was a long check-in line. The office was filled with applicants, many physically disabled in wheelchairs. It was depressing.

Was I now considered seriously disabled like these people?

After about thirty minutes in line, I reached the check-in desk. My head began to hurt. More paperwork. I took a seat and waited another hour until I was called. I followed a clerk into what looked like a glorified office cubby.

"Hello, my name is Dr. McBride," said a heavy-set woman in a floral dress behind a small desk. "Please have a seat."

She looked at the intake sheet. "Mrs. Helm. What is your complaint?"

It was right there on the top line. Whatever.

I quickly relayed to her why I was there and told her about the persistent double vision that prevented me from working.

"How did you get this condition?"

"I was in a car accident about a year ago. I had a concussion."

"I see. Any memory loss?"

"Not really."

"You mean you haven't experienced some memory loss?"

"A little. Nothing serious."

"Good. Then the tests won't take too long. These cognitive tests are standard in cases involving concussions. Let's begin."

She asked me to name the current president, to count backward by sevens from 100, and to recall items from a list she read to me after several minutes. Next came several tests that required me to read words or look at shapes on a piece of paper. My eyes were getting tired.

"How much more of this do I have to do?"

"We have at least another hour. Do you need a break?"

"Yes. I'm not sure my eyes will be able to take another hour of this."

"Take as many breaks as you need."

Although I did my best to power through, I left the session feeling dizzy and nauseous. My double vision and frustration escalated as a result of having to jump through yet another hoop. The sunlight seemed overly bright, and I had to squint as I returned to the car.

"How'd it go?" Jade asked as I got into the car.

"Who knows? They said I'd get the results in six to eight weeks."

"Wow, how were the tests?"

"They were grueling. My head hurts, and my double vision is bad. I will be worthless for doing any driving, reading, or thinking the rest of the day. I hate this!"

"I am sorry, Mom."

"It is wrong to give me these tests with my vision issues. It's like asking someone in a wheelchair to run a mile."

Jade nodded in agreement.

The next morning, still depressed over the experience, I puttered around the house aimlessly, trying to complete a few chores. Remembering that I would need to go through more testing for the lawsuit, I wondered if I had the stamina to move

CHICKEN THERAPY

forward. I fled outside to find relief, remembering I had not yet let the chickens out of the coop.

A few minutes after the rowdy flock left the run, Orloff wandered out of the coop and bumped into me. She then loudly jumped to the side and squawked as if insulted that I had just bumped into her. Scurrying to keep up with the rest of the flock, she headed to the brick steps where the rest of the chickens had already athletically descended to forage in the yard below.

I stopped to watch her as she positioned both feet side by side with her long toes curled over the edge of the top step. After a pause, she focused on the next step, spread her wings, and wildly leaped to the step below until she got to the bottom. It was obvious that she still suffered from the injury she had sustained the day we found her injured, lifeless body at the bottom of the hill. She had found a way to cope.

I decided that my new goal was to have a better attitude and perspective on life, to find ways to live with my condition, and not be victimized by it or let it drag me down.

At the grocery store, I tried to remember to ask the clerks how their day was going rather than just hurrying out of the store. They sometimes seemed surprised that someone took time out of their busy day to even notice them.

At home, phone calls from creditors and bill collectors had once been irritating and confrontational. Now, I found a way to turn them into negotiating sessions that were mediated through kindness and respect. I made peace with the world and found it in myself.

******

At my next visit with Dr. Monroe, he reported that my vision was not stabilizing or getting better, even with my new eye exercises.

It wasn't news to me.

"It looks like surgery won't be an option."

"Isn't there anything else you can do?"

"Not unless something changes. You might need to get used to your new normal."

I could do nothing but nod in agreement as I choked back the sobs that were involuntarily welling up. I didn't want to accept that I would never be able to get my old life back.

As the weeks passed, I no longer had the strength or desire to pursue a positive attitude. Time, something I once never had enough of, now seemed to drag on in an endless routine, depending on how my vision was each day. The bills were continuing to mount up. I checked the mailbox every day for word from Social Security.

Finally, one day the letter arrived. I opened the envelope and skipped through all the jargon about the tests and procedures to read the final line in bold:

Your application for Social Security disability insurance has been denied.

My heart sank. I called Jon.

"I can't believe it. After all the BS you've gone through."

"What should we do?"

"Call Henry. See what he says."

I hung up and made myself a cup of tea, then called Henry, expecting to get his voicemail. Surprisingly, he picked up. I explained the situation.

"I'm sorry. It's what happens most of the time with Social Security."

"It doesn't make any sense. I can't work because of my injury. All the tests and my doctors' records confirm it."

"Well, you can appeal. It takes time, but it's an option."

"Can you help with that?"

"I'm afraid not. I am a personal injury lawyer. You need a Social Security disability lawyer to represent you." He paused a moment. "I know just the guy. His name is Carl Steinway. He's not far from you."

After some brief research, I found out that what Henry had said was right. On average, over 63% of the applications received are denied. To move forward, those applicants must appeal and attend a hearing. Hiring an SSD lawyer is the best way to obtain acceptance at the appeal.

I contacted Carl and explained my situation.

"I guess I just don't understand why I have to work so hard at proving to them that I can't work."

"Yes, it is overly complicated. That's just how the system works, unfortunately. I can help you with the appeal if you like."

"How long will that take?"

"Probably a few months."

Months! "Why so long?"

"The system is bogged down. I have represented people who have had terminal cancer. Some have passed by the time they receive any compensation. It's a crying shame."

"I guess I have no choice but to try. How does it work?"

He explained that once we sign a contract, he will file for an appeal immediately.

"I would need you to get me as many medical records as possible."

"How much will it cost?"

"If we're successful, my fee will be one-third of all the retroactive amounts you receive. If we are not, there is no cost to you."

"Okay. I'll speak with my husband and get back to you."

"That's highway robbery," Jon said later that evening.

"I know. I looked it up. It's the standard fee. I crunched some numbers and I think it will be worth it if we win."

"I guess it is worth a shot."

CHICKEN THERAPY

I called Carl and had him send the contract overnight. That made two law cases we had to endure with no end in sight.

A few mornings later, after breakfast, I meandered out to the coop and opened the run door. The chickens clamored out, the dominant ones pecking at the docile ones, to ensure their high-ranking position of first chicken out the door. The sounds of flailing wings and shrieking cackles filled the air as the cavalcade greeted the morning. The ducks followed, clumsily waddling behind with their loud, bossy quacks.

The young ducks then raced across the dewy grass, pummeling the air with their wings, as they attempted to become airborne. The older ducks, now way too fat to fly, also did a run, just to show the young ones they could if they really wanted to. I knew they couldn't, and it made me chuckle.

A few hens would observe the show and then also do a wild run, hoping that maybe today was the day they too would fly. They all tried every day, not caring if they failed. Failing to survive was their only concern. *Could I find a way to embrace each new day, not caring if I failed the day before? What if accepting the new me isn't failing? Maybe I have this all wrong.*

For the next few days, I wrote in my journal about the experiences I had with Social Security, making sure to take plenty of breaks. I wrote about all the doctors, and my most recent debilitating visit to Dr. Monroe. I wrote about the lessons gleaned from my flock. As I wrote, I realized that I had been looking for a magic bullet cure for my condition from a whole series of so-called specialists.

It was clear they couldn't help me. Maybe I had to look outside the medical community. Maybe there was another avenue I had overlooked. I had no idea where to start.

I thought about Anita, my concussion therapist. Of all the medical professionals I had seen, she had been the most pleasant

CHICKEN THERAPY

and caring, understanding, and hopeful. Even though it had been a long time since we worked together, maybe she could advise me.

I found her number and, with a deep breath, made the call. Relieved that I reached her voicemail and with my voice shaking, I introduced myself and asked her to return my call. I was pleasantly surprised when she called a few hours later.

"Hi, Chris. How are the chickens?"

"Thanks for calling me back. I wasn't sure you'd remember me. They're all fine." I paused, surprised that she not only remembered me but remembered that I had chickens.

"I'm not."

"What's happening?"

Hesitantly, I briefly tried to describe the saga of the medical care I had received in the past year and a half. "Sounds like you've been through the mill."

"That's an understatement. I was wondering if you had any suggestions for some other approach."

She thought for a moment. "Has anyone recommended VT?"

"VT?"

"Vision Therapy."

Thinking back, I remembered that I had had some experience with vision therapy with Jade and her ADD when she was little. It had been successful.

"Isn't it just for kids? I remember it helped my daughter with her ADD when she was young."

"It's not just for kids. While vision therapy can help children with learning difficulties, it can also benefit adults with a variety of vision problems."

"Even if my nerves were damaged from the concussion?"

"It won't cure the damage, but it could help you manage your double vision and other symptoms."

"If it can be so effective, why didn't any of the doctors recommend it?"

"Medical doctors aren't taught about vision therapy in medical school. Mostly optometrists know about it, but it requires additional training to make it part of their practice, so they don't take the time."

"Thanks. I'll check it out. I don't remember the person who helped my daughter, it's been so long ago. Do you know anyone in the area?"

She gave me the names of a few optometrists who specialize in vision therapy. "Good luck and stay in touch. Let me know if it helps."

"I will. Thank you so much."

Jon and I spent the next few days doing as much research online about vision therapy as possible. Vision therapy is a program of specifically sequenced activities, including the use of lenses, filters, and prisms, designed to develop, improve, or remediate functional visual skills, visual perception, and visual-motor integration.

There seem to have been hundreds of published research studies showing the effectiveness of vision therapy. However, it was still considered an alternative or complementary protocol. It is not endorsed by the American Medical Association, the American Academy of Ophthalmology, the Mayo Clinic, the American Orthoptic Council, and the American Association of Pediatric Ophthalmology and Strabismus. Maybe that was the reason most doctors do not recommend it. Only the AOA, the American Optometric Association, has advocated for vision therapy as a viable and effective practice.

Hoping that VT might be a viable approach, Jon looked at the website of one of the offices, Vision Therapy Associates, that Anita recommended.

"Christa Roser, O.D., FCOVD is the director and has extensive qualifications. So do the other optometrists on staff. I would give them a call."

CHICKEN THERAPY

I quickly scanned the website.

"They mention concussion, traumatic brain injury, and strabismus on the front page. Sounds promising."

The next day, I called. After a brief conversation with Sara, the receptionist, she told me that I sounded like a good candidate for vision therapy and that she could set me up for an evaluation next week."

"Do you take insurance?"

"We do participate with insurance companies. Check to see if it's covered by your company. If so, we will submit the paperwork for you. Many insurance companies will reimburse you part of the fee."

Sara sounded so nice and honest that I decided to go for it.

"Okay. See you next week."

While I tried to temper my expectations, I was hopeful that this could be a path to help me take more control of my life. I called the insurance company and asked about coverage. My school insurance had run out, and we were now on Jon's insurance. The woman on the phone was pleasant while she informed me that they didn't cover "that type of therapy." Disappointed, I decided if it worked, it would be worth the additional expense.

The office of Vision Therapy Associates was fifteen daunting miles of freeways and traffic away. Jon had to drive me. It was a good day, and my vision was not that bad. When we arrived, he parked close to the entrance.

"I will be here if you need me." He was used to my need to go to appointments myself.

Upon entering the cheery office, I noticed that the people waiting were either seniors or children with their mothers. Like Jade and I had been decades ago. I felt a bit uncomfortable and out of place, as I was not part of either group.

I checked in with Sara.

"Hi, Chris, nice to meet you." She handed me a few forms to fill out.

I shakily sat down, reached for my purse to retrieve my reading glasses, and struggled to read through the material. Thankfully, they were the usual general health questions with yes and no answers. Before I could finish filling out the forms, Sara called my name. "I'm not done with the forms."

"That's okay. You can finish them later."

I dutifully followed a young man into the next room where I took a seat in the all-too-familiar ophthalmic chair. A few minutes later, the optometrist walked in.

"Hi, Chris. I'm Dr. Roser. I'll need to conduct a few tests, so please make yourself comfortable."

Dr. Roser was dressed casually in corduroy pants and a blouse with horses on it. She was a small, confident woman with short hair and wire-rimmed glasses. I liked her immediately.

Numb to the process by now, I just sat there. Once the tests were completed, Dr. Roser reviewed the results and explained them to me. They were all too familiar: cranial nerve damage, eye movement challenges, and double vision. It was déjà vu, and I was sick of hearing it. I thought it would be different somehow.

"I've heard it all before. It's frustrating. Nothing has helped."

She nodded. "I know it's hard. To avoid double vision, you have unknowingly stopped moving your eyes in any direction that makes you see double. That is why the temporary damage to the sixth cranial nerve is not getting better. It is from lack of use. We see this all the time in victims of traumatic brain injury, particularly from car accidents."

This was new. It was the first time any doctor explained the origins of the problem so clearly. She did not talk at me; she talked to me.

"Oh? You see this all the time?"

"Yes, it is not infrequent, but I've got some good news. We can help you regain the use of your sixth cranial nerve. However, the nerve palsy of your fourth cranial nerve is permanent. It impedes normal eye movement, causing you to see double."

"I'm not sure I understand. Does that mean you can cure it?"

"Not quite, although it is treatable. We will teach you how to exercise the muscles controlled by the sixth cranial nerve. Then we will work with you to train your brain to understand the images it receives. Your double vision should improve slowly over the course of the treatment. It will be hard work, with lots of practice at home. Once we're through, you should be able to manage your condition quite well."

I wanted to believe her, to hope for a normal future.

"How does it work?"

"Each weekly session lasts around an hour. We keep it short to avoid eye fatigue. We give you exercises to do at home between each visit. We'll monitor your progress throughout the treatment and make any adjustments necessary to the program."

"How long do you think it will take?"

"It's hard to tell. Given your nerve damage and experiences over the past few years, it may take at least six months."

I panicked inside. *How will we ever be able to afford this?* Then I realized that this was the first ray of hope I'd received. If it could possibly work, then I'd find a way.

"Thank you. This is the best news I have received in a long time."

"I'm glad," she said, smiling. "Remember it's not a 'cure.' It's a method of relieving your symptoms and putting you in control of your vision."

"I understand. That's all I want."

"Great. See you next week then. Thanks for coming in."

CHICKEN THERAPY

After booking my appointment schedule, I left feeling full of renewed hope for the future.

On the drive home, I explained to Jon what had just occurred. "The big difference between today's exam and the others was the compassionate way the staff listened to my story about my vision challenges. They treated me like a normal person who had come seeking help. Not a lost cause victim."

"If it's that easy, why didn't any of your doctors recommend it?"

The optometrist said that although they get occasional referrals from medical doctors, including neurologists, concussion specialists, and ophthalmologists, many doctors just don't know how it works, what it is, or what it can do. So, maybe it's pretty much off their radar."

Jon nodded thoughtfully. "It'll take a minimum of six months and will put a strain on our budget."

"Don't worry. If there's a chance it will help you, we have to take it. You'll know if it's working before that."

I loved him for his ability to simplify these situations with unwavering support. He looked at most challenges as problems to be solved, not as excuses for giving up.

The lamp post stands there,

Tall and proud,

Never moving, never loud,

It has one job, to light the lawn,

Turn on at dusk, turn off at dawn.

CHAPTER 20

My appointments were set up around Jade's schedule so she could drive me to the VT office for at least the first month. I hoped that by then, I might be feeling well enough to drive myself. She was happy to oblige.

The first therapy appointment seemed a bit odd to me. It was in a room of cubicles down the hall past the exam offices, filled with what appeared to be elementary school-type materials. I could hear the conversations of the other therapists and patients around me and wondered how I could ever concentrate.

"Please have a seat," the attendant said as we stopped at a cubicle. "Evelyn will be with you shortly."

Evelyn? I thought that Dr. Roser would be conducting the treatment.

A few minutes later, I met Evelyn. She was about my age, well-dressed with long blonde hair and a friendly smile.

"Hi, Chris. I'm Evelyn Mosco. I'll be your therapist."

"Hi. Where's Dr. Roser?"

"Dr. Roser does all the initial testing. I'm the VT therapist."

"How long have you been a vision therapist?"

"Since I graduated from Shippensburg."

"Shippensburg University? I graduated from Shippensburg!"

As the discussion progressed, we figured out that she had graduated a few years before me and that we had both rented the same house in our senior year. That connection helped me feel even more comfortable.

"Okay, tell me more about your double vision."

"I've had double vision since my car accident several years ago. It is usually the worst when I get tired. I tried prism glasses, but they didn't help much."

"Is there a particularly bad sight line?"

"Yes. On the left."

She made a note. "How is your vision today?"

"Not too bad."

"Good. We'll begin with simple exercises. Be sure to let me know if you get tired, and we'll take a break."

That was a relief. A therapist who understood.

She had me look in different directions, not focusing on anything. It was difficult at first, but she said they would get easier with practice.

Next, I was introduced to eye stretches. I had to cover one eye, move it as far to the left as I could, and hold it for 10 seconds. I then moved the same eye up, then down, and to the right. I did the same with the other eye. It felt sort of like stretching my body in yoga class. It made me realize just how tight my eye muscles were.

"I started doing something like this a few months earlier. It seemed to help."

"Yes, your eye muscles are tight from lack of use. Are you okay to continue?"

"I'm fine."

Next, she had me look at a stick a few inches from my nose and then look at a sticker on the wall.

"This exercise will help you learn to focus from near to far," she explained. "Does anything look double?"

"The stick."

"Okay. Now relax your eyes and look at the stick."

I had no idea what that meant, tried to just calm down, and then focus on the stick. Miraculously, I saw one image.

"It's single."

"Good. Now, look at the sticker on the wall."

As I shifted my eyes to the wall, I felt that familiar physical pain around my eye and immediately saw double. I stopped and explained what happened. She calmly said to try again.

It happened again. My face felt hot, and I could feel my anxiety increase.

"Don't worry. It takes time. Take a minute, then try again."

I tried but to no avail.

"Are you feeling nauseous? Dizzy?"

"A little."

"Okay. Let's take a five-minute break." She reached into a drawer, took out some hard candies, and handed them to me. "These are ginger candies. When you feel nauseous from the exercises, take a break and eat one. It will help."

This was new. I had always relied on butter mints. Sure enough, within a few minutes of popping one of the sweet candies in my mouth, I felt much better. The ginger was much more effective.

Evelyn then showed me a simple exercise that would relax my aching eyes and relieve the dizziness.

"Gently cup your hands over your eyes, relax, close your eyes, and concentrate on the dark for a minute or so."

I did.

"Okay, take your hands away."

To my amazement, that simple trick caused a lot of the pain and dizziness to disappear.

"Better?"

"Much."

"Now let's try the focus exercises again."

It was still difficult, but at least I didn't feel sick.

Next, she took out a few cards. "Let's play a visual memory game."

Remembering the horrible experience with the psychologist, I hesitated. "My memory's fine."

"Your memory does not just involve your brain. It also involves your eyes as well. Your eyes see the picture and then your brain stores it. Some of this process has been disrupted due to your

CHICKEN THERAPY

injuries. We need to reteach your brain how to process these images."

At first, I felt a little stupid and embarrassed because the game was exactly like the memory game I played with my children when they were very young. The cards in this game were bigger and there were fewer of them. It didn't take me long to figure out that Evelyn was right. It was more of a challenge than I thought it would be.

We played three times. I was ecstatic when I improved my score on the last try, and it didn't make me feel sick.

"Great job! I didn't think you were going to be able to find the other rooster," Evelyn said while putting away the cards.

"Hen."

"Hen?"

"The chicken is a hen, not a rooster."

"How can you tell?" Evelyn said.

"I have chickens. Roosters are bigger and usually have larger combs on their heads and red fleshy wattles that hang down from their faces."

"How many do you have? Do you eat them?"

"No. I do eat chicken. These are more pets to me than farm animals. We do get lots of eggs, though."

Evelyn sat intently, listening to me explain the dynamics of having a flock of chickens.

"Our time is up for today. This is my lunch break, so we can go a few minutes over," she said, glancing at her watch. "It sounds like you enjoy raising these chickens!"

"I do. Now that my life has slowed down, I take the time to observe them. I find them fascinating. I feel normal when I am with them."

"Sounds like they are good therapy."

"Yes. Chicken therapy!"

Evelyn chuckled. "I am so glad that you are learning to find joy in everyday life. That's what I have found to be my patients' biggest obstacle after a life-changing event."

She gave me a folder with instructions on some of the exercises I had done during the session.

"I want you to try to do these three times a day at home. You may have to work up to that. Do as many as you can. Don't push it. If you start having symptoms, just stop. If your symptoms do not go away in twenty minutes, you know you have done too much."

"Will do."

"You'll also find a handout about some lifestyle suggestions, such as tips on diet, resting, and how to do daily activities to avoid symptoms."

"Thanks. This is useful. I often overdo."

"Number one rule: Be kind to yourself. Get the rest you need."

"I'll try. What about reading or computer work?"

"Can you read for 20 minutes?"

"I think so. I never really kept track of the time."

"Well, you need to do it now. Set a timer."

"Like for the wash?"

"Yes, that'll work. Then follow the 20-20-20 rule."

"What's that?"

"It's pretty simple. 20 minutes on the computer, reading a book, looking at your phone, or other close-up work. Then look at something 20 feet away for at least 20 seconds before returning to it. If the symptoms continue, move on to some other activity that doesn't involve focusing so close."

"That might be tough."

"It doesn't need to be precise. Keep a record of when symptoms occur and what might bring them on so we can work on continuing the same activity for longer periods."

I listened intently to her advice. It all made sense.

CHICKEN THERAPY

"Also, do not plan more than one stressful activity each day. Things like coming to vision therapy or a doctor's appointment, even socializing with friends, and long shopping trips are all stressful to your brain and eyes. We will help you get to the point where doing multiple activities in one day gets easier. For now, you need to set limits."

"Got it."

"Any questions?"

"No. I think I've got it. Thanks for your help."

"Okay. See you next week. Good luck."

It was the first time I left a medical office feeling motivated, not depressed.

"You look happy," Jade said as I got into the car.

"I am. This could help."

"How's the therapist?"

"Her name is Evelyn and she was great."

Jade dropped me off at home and went to her class. I collapsed on the couch for a three-hour nap. Evelyn's Number One rule: Get the rest I need. When I woke up, I sat down with a cup of tea and browsed through the literature Evelyn had given me. It was written in a simple, clear, easy-to-read format. All the information was practical and helpful.

The next day after breakfast and tending to my flock, I sat down, took out my vision therapy folder, and began the first exercise, determined to make this work. I looked at the pencil in front of me and then at a Post-it note I had placed on the wall. It was double. After only a few minutes, I felt some slight symptoms.

"Take a break," I reminded myself.

After closing my eyes, cupping the palm of my hands over my eyes, and resting for a few minutes, I tried again. I looked at the Post-it note until it became single and then back at the pencil. Now the pencil was double.

"Try it again," I could hear Evelyn saying in my head.

The third time was the charm. The pencil became single. I quickly moved on to the next exercise, energized and happy with my small victory. After the third exercise, I felt nauseous, and my eyes hurt. I stopped and ate a ginger candy. Maybe I should try the other two in the middle of the day, I decided, and put the folder away.

I eventually figured out a good routine. I would take an hour each morning to alternate the eye exercises and a few body stretches, followed by some light physical therapy exercises. Then I did half of the eye exercises again after lunch and the other half after dinner. The time between sessions gave my eyes enough rest to avoid symptoms and to take care of my other chores.

Later that week, I headed outside to do some yard work. Lady Gaga was racing through the weeds nearby, navigating past the rest of the flock with ease. When we first got her as a chick, she could get around just fine. Once her crest completely grew in, she began to have difficulty entering the coop and finding a roost, especially once the sun went down. Her crest feather impeded her vision.

Watching her weave through the yard now without bumping into anything, I realized that she had developed a system that worked for her to manage her vision issue. Her head feathers presented obstacles to her daily life, and she learned to cope. With vision therapy, I could do the same.

Every now and then the bulb burns out,

Yet the lamp post stands there proudly,

It does not scream or shout.

CHAPTER 21

As the weeks progressed, I looked forward to my sessions with Evelyn. They were helping immensely but were exhausting. When I had a hard time with an exercise, she never made me feel like a failure. I was grateful for that.

"Try this," Evelyn said as she handed me a coin. "Hold the coin eye level at arm's length. Look at it for five seconds. Now hold it as high above your head as you can and look at it for five seconds. Next, hold it at your waist and look at it for five seconds."

As soon as I looked down and tried to focus on the coin, it was blurry. I felt dizzy and felt myself sway.

"Let's take a break and try again in a few minutes. Take some deep breaths. Have a ginger drop."

I sat down on the chair and rested my eyes, determined to be able to do this.

"Okay, let's start over."

I tried. "Still dizzy," I said, "and the coin isn't blurry!"

"Great! Now do it again."

"I don't think I can!"

"I know it is hard. One more time."

I did. The coin was still blurry.

"Okay, let's move on. You'll like this next exercise. This is a fun way to work on getting back some of your peripheral vision."

She led me to a room that contained a large board approximately six feet wide and four feet high. It reminded me of a blackboard in a classroom, only it was covered with many large plastic buttons. The goal of the exercise was to hit each button with my hand when it lit up, like the Whack-a-Mole game. The catch was that I had to look at the center of the board and, without moving my head, touch each button as it lit up on the board.

The board was hooked up to a computer that would keep score of the number of buttons I could accurately hit. The game immediately improved my mood as my competitive nature surfaced. I smiled as I scrambled to hit the buttons, improving each time.

Another exercise was Wall Ball. It was one of my favorites. At first, I just had to throw a small rubber ball against the wall while looking at one spot, and then catch it on the rebound. When I eventually mastered that, I had to read a chart with letters on it — while throwing and catching the ball.

I was also given exercises to improve my balance. I had to stand on one foot while using the other foot to trace figure eights in the air. First to the right, then in front, and then behind me. The hardest balance exercise was the tree pose, a yoga position. It required me to put the sole of my foot against a thigh while putting my hands above my head in a prayer position and then to hold that position.

"Remember to breathe when doing these and always have a chair nearby to use in case you need additional support."

At the end of this session, Evelyn told me to stop by Dr. Roser's office to pick up some paperwork.

"How are you, Chris?" Dr. Roser said as she handed me an envelope.

"Getting better. Evelyn is terrific."

"Good to hear. Your lawyer, Henry Arsdale, asked me to write an evaluation of my findings for your lawsuit. He is also giving them to your Social Security lawyer. Here is a copy."

"Thank you. This is all so overwhelming. The test Social Security made me go through was torture. I have to go through more testing for the lawsuit."

"I am so sorry. We see this a lot. If it is any help, we have noticed that the stress and testing they put you through make recovering difficult. We're here to help you get through it. Once it is all over, many patients improve more rapidly."

"That is good to hear."

"Most people have no idea how grueling it is to deal with insurance companies, government agencies, and lawsuits after a car accident. You are constantly reminded of your issues, never able to get a break from it… and all those tests only make it worse."

***

Each session usually began with Evelyn inquiring about my week. One day, when I explained that going into grocery stores still made me feel disoriented and dizzy, she led me into a room to try a new exercise.

"Walk a straight line from here to the wall. When you take a step with your left foot, turn your head to the left and focus on something on the wall. When you take a step with your right foot, turn your head to the right and do the same."

As I did as she instructed, I was surprised at how hard it was to perform those simple tasks fluidly.

"Why aren't you turning your head to the left?" Evelyn inquired.

"That is as far as it turns now."

"Really? Well, that can be affecting your vision. Your brain and eyes are expecting your head to look further left. When it doesn't, your brain must readjust to the signals it receives."

"I am not sure how to do that."

"When you turn your head, focus your eye on what you see. Look at it until it comes into focus. I know it's a lot. I will put this on your list of home exercises."

Vision therapy was the first place that took into consideration how all my injuries potentially played a role in my symptoms. They treated the whole person, not just the eyes. All the specialists

CHICKEN THERAPY

I had seen concentrated on a specific problem, but never seemed to connect how each injury might be affecting another. Evelyn made this insane world I was now a part of seem a little less scary.

During one session, I explained to her that I was writing a journal and sheepishly told her that it seemed easier writing in large letters with crayon on an artist's pad.

"Wow, that is a great idea! The letters you write in crayons are bigger and bolder than words written in pencil or pen. I'll pass that along to my other patients."

As the weeks passed, the vision therapy sessions finally gave me a place to go where I felt like I fit in. I realized that I did not seek the solace of the coop as my retreat as much as I used to. Although I still enjoyed being with my flock and observing their antics, I was slowly feeling more comfortable with my life away from them.

You see, the lamp post had decided long ago,

Not to worry about what it cannot control,

The lamp post stands there tall and proud,

Knowing that a new bulb will appear,

Even if it doesn't know how.

CHAPTER 22

Two months later, I had my first evaluation since my original exam at Vision Therapy Associates. Giddy with excitement, I pulled into the parking lot. My vision had improved to the point that I could now drive myself. I had done the home exercises every day and followed all the advice Evelyn had given me. I even looked forward to going through the tests and felt confident that they would show my progress.

After the testing, Dr. Roser smiled. "I'm happy to report that you have regained the use of the sixth cranial nerve in both eyes. Your vision is not back to normal but much improved."

"Does that mean that my vision will improve even more?"

"Yes, I believe so. Evelyn says you are a model patient. I recommend you continue for the next three months."

I readily agreed to continue the program despite the cost. Anything that would get me closer to my old life was worth it.

******

Meanwhile, our finances were still precarious. I was still waiting for some word about my appeal to Social Security. After leaving several messages, Carl called back to say that he had received the notice that my Social Security disability appeal hearing was set for 10:00 a.m. on the Thursday of the following week.

I was concerned we had only a few days to prepare. For something this important, it all seemed so haphazard.

"Don't worry. It always happens this way."

"What do I need to bring?"

"Nothing. The judge has all the relevant material. Meet me at the Social Security office in Harrisburg about 30 minutes before the hearing so we can prepare."

CHICKEN THERAPY

"What is the address?"

"I will send you the information in an email. It is near the Capitol building. Parking can be tough, so consider that when planning your drive time."

That night I told Jon that the hearing was three days away.

"And you were only informed today? Don't these people realize we have lives? How can they expect us to just drop everything because they're so disorganized?"

"I know. Carl says that's the way the system is. Hopefully, it'll be over soon, and we'll get some relief."

I tried to sound optimistic, while on the inside, I was panicking. *What happens if they deny our appeal? Would we have to tighten our already stressed budget? Would I have to stop my vision therapy just as it was getting me back to a life I could feel proud of?* That night, I had a hard time sleeping. I went downstairs to the darkened kitchen and looked out into the night.

A black cloud suddenly emerged in the ring of a faintly lit sky that surrounded the full moon. It reminded me of a black cloud I had seen in a nightmare when I was a little girl. Back then, I had been afraid and overwhelmed by a sense of doom. It sent chills down my spine to remember that feeling. Was it some harbinger about tomorrow's hearing?

I thought about all my blessings: my family; my flock; my overall health. The fact that I was seeing better every day. I just needed more time to heal and get back to a semblance of a normal life. I had to remain grateful for the progress I was making.

I looked past the dark cloud into the soft light of the moon and prayed for help, for peace, and for acceptance of whatever might happen tomorrow. I whispered the Lord's Prayer, ending with a deeply felt *Amen*. I felt calmer, letting go of my fear and anxiety with faith in God's will. I went back to bed and slept.

CHICKEN THERAPY

I awoke the next day refreshed, resigned that I would accept whatever the day would bring. When we arrived at the office in Harrisburg, I realized that, ironically, it was near the building that housed the Harrisburg University of Science and Technology. I remembered my visit there before starting my master's degree, the degree I would never obtain. It made my stomach knot. The accident had taken so much from me.

Jon and I arrived at the Social Security office and ascended to the eighth floor, where we were greeted by a security officer. He searched my purse and then scanned us with a wand. We were then instructed to sit in the waiting room with several other people until my name was called.

"Where's Carl?" Jon asked. "Shouldn't he be here by now?"

"He said he'd meet us here. I'll call him."

Just as I was about to dial, a man in a shabby suit with a briefcase walked up to us.

"Chris Helm?"

"Yes."

"Carl Steinway."

"I was getting a bit worried. Nice to meet you." We shook hands. "This is my husband, Jon."

"Sorry, the traffic was bad. Good to have you both here. We've got a few minutes before the hearing. Let's go to the conference room, and I'll explain the process." He led us into a conference room.

Although I had never met him face to face, he came recommended by Henry. The few conversations we had on the phone and his website led me to believe he was experienced in this kind of appeal. We sat at a worn wooden table as he took out a manila folder from his briefcase.

"First off, the judge will ask you to explain why you can't work. Then a vocational expert will ask you a few questions concerning your job and the challenges your condition presents. Let's go over what you will say."

As he went over the kinds of questions I might be asked, I was concerned that even though I had explained my condition and sent Carl my medical records, he did not seem to understand my condition or how it prevented me from working. I started to feel anxious that the judge might not also.

"You might be asked about your attempts to resolve your medical disability." He looked at the file. "I see some notes about the special glasses and medication."

"Yes, none of it helped."

"I see you are currently being treated with vision therapy. What does that involve? It's first for—"

Before I could answer, a clerk knocked on the door to let us know that the judge was ready for us.

"Don't worry. Just answer as concisely as possible."

Jon was told to remain outside in the waiting area.

"Good luck," he said and squeezed my hand.

They and I were escorted to a large, brightly lit conference room. In the middle was a big U-shaped table that was capped on the end by an elevated podium. A clerk instructed Carl and me where to sit.

The judge was seated at the podium. His black robe, stern appearance, and position above the rest of the room were intimidating. I wondered if that was intentional. To his left, at the end of the table sat a spindly poorly dressed court stenographer.

To his right on the other side of the table was another woman whom I assumed was the vocational expert. I tried not to look at her as she was in my field of double vision. I closed my eyes for a few seconds to calm down.

The judge opened the proceeding by introducing himself, stating the date and time, and the name of the occupational expert.

CHICKEN THERAPY

Carl introduced himself and me. Then, without looking directly at me, the judge explained the proceedings for the record and commented that my disability case was unique in his experience.

Not the best way to begin.

At that moment, I realized that adults with head injuries like mine, who appear normal and speak normally, simply were not on the court's radar as qualifying for disability insurance. As much as I hated being labeled "disabled," the fact that my injuries prevented me from returning to my career made me as eligible as anyone to get the financial assistance.

The judge asked a few simple informational questions about my previous employment and the accident. He seemed fair and compassionate. At one point, he mentioned that although he saw the diagnoses made by several specialists, he did not see a list of symptoms and restrictions that made me unable to work. He only had notes from the neuro-ophthalmologist and an optometrist saying that I was unable to perform my current job. He asked my attorney if he had this information.

"I thought it was in the documentation, Your Honor. I can get it to the court shortly if it is deemed necessary."

Why hadn't he known that this was needed? I had asked him if I needed to bring any of my records. He said the court had everything needed. I sat there feeling my case was doomed.

The judge ignored him. "In the interest of time, Mrs. Helm, please state your symptoms and explain why this court should grant you compensation?"

I froze. It all came down to me now.

"My concussion caused severe damage to my cranial nerves. As a result, I have double vision, dizziness, nausea, headaches, and lack of peripheral vision. These conditions prevent me from working as a teacher and an educational tech specialist because I am unable to use a computer or read or engage in classroom instruction for sustained periods. I cannot work at any job that requires these activities."

"Can you explain to me what a day in your life is like now?" the judge asked, trying to clarify what I had just explained.

Pausing for a moment, I tried to think how to best explain.

"I stay at home mostly. I can do chores and make short trips to the grocery store or doctor's appointments. I can't read or work on a computer for more than a few minutes at a time."

"Can you drive?" the judge asked.

"Yes, but only recently and only for short distances to familiar places. I can't negotiate heavy traffic or highways. I find it hard to read road signs. I can't drive at night."

"I see. Do you have double vision now in this room?"

"Yes. The double vision is always present when I look to the left, and as the day goes on, or if I do too many activities. As my eyes get tired, my vision becomes blurry or double when I look straight on."

I took a deep breath and summed up my case.

"I lost my job because I couldn't keep up with the demands of teaching and computer work. I need some kind of compensation to make up for my job loss."

"Thank you, Mrs. Helm. I think I understand."

"Your Honor," the vocational expert said, "I have a question."

"Proceed."

"Mrs. Helm, I see you are being treated with vision therapy. Will it resolve your condition?"

"Unfortunately, no. At least not completely. It can't undo the cranial nerve damage. Vision therapy helps me manage my symptoms, and helps my brain better understand what it sees. I will always have the challenges that prevent me from working as a teacher."

"Your Honor," Carl said. "My client has done an excellent job explaining her situation. Her previous employment record

CHICKEN THERAPY

and the medical documentation all indicate that she was a very hardworking teacher who is no longer capable of performing this or any other full-time job."

"Yes, I can see that, Mr. Steinway."

The hearing concluded with the judge saying that I would receive notice of the final decision regarding my appeal in a few weeks. Then, he ended the session and called for the next case. That was our cue to leave the room.

"That seemed to go well," Carl said in the hall.

"I hope so. Why weren't my symptoms in the file?" I asked.

"I thought that the diagnosis from your doctors and their notes would be enough. Your testimony fulfilled the requirement. The judge seemed to understand the issue. It'll probably go your way."

"Probably?"

"The judge seemed sympathetic, but as he stated, it is an unusual case. It all seemed positive though."

"I hope you're right."

"I'll be in touch as soon as I get the judgment."

I stormed out of the building with Jon in tow. I was furious.

"Sounds like it didn't go well," Jon said.

"Carl didn't file the right paperwork. The judge was nice enough to give me a chance to explain the problem. I think he got it. We'll know in a few weeks. I'm exhausted. Let's go home."

I wish I had the courage,

To join the others in the play,

To try out for a part,

Instead of waiting for that day.

CHAPTER 23

At my next vision therapy session, I told Evelyn about the hearing and my vision issues.

"I understand. Stress can bring back the symptoms. I'm sure things will go your way. Let's get started."

Although my double vision, peripheral vision, and symptoms were all improved, they were still there. Many of the therapy sessions were still very difficult. When I mastered one exercise, Evelyn always gave me another, more difficult task to replace it.

"No rest for the weary!" Evelyn said light-heartedly when I got particularly frustrated. She always found a way to push me while understanding the emotional toll from the fallout of the accident that I carried.

Probably one of the most important but difficult exercises involved a computer. I had to stand a few feet from a computer screen wearing a pair of special non-prescription glasses that had a red lens in one eye and green in the other.

"How do these work?" I curiously asked while putting them on.

"They make your eyes work together. Although the pictures look black and white on the screen, they have stripes of red and green in them. The eye with the red lens can't see what's under the green film, so the other eye must see it. Another part of the picture has a green stripe so the eye with the red lens can't see it. Both eyes need to work together for you to be able to see the entire picture clearly."

"I understand."

"Look at the first picture. What do you see?"

The computer screen showed a picture of a person or an animal and many background objects such as trees or houses. It was hard to make everything come into focus.

CHICKEN THERAPY

The harder I tried, the more double the sketch became. Then something weird happened.

"It's not working. I think one eye is only seeing black, like it turned off or something."

"Your brain is ignoring the visual signal of that eye. It can't figure out the image, so it is trying to adapt. Let's take a break."

I sat at Evelyn's desk and sucked on a ginger hard candy for my nausea.

"Let's try this. Rest your elbows on the table, close your eyes, and cup your hands over them. They are tired because they are constantly taking in new visual information and sending it to your brain to be processed. Your brain is also tired. It is working hard."

Evelyn's explanations always made me feel confident and informed. For the past two years, I rarely understood why I felt tired and irritable trying to do normal activities. Doctors either spoke in technical jargon or ignored my concerns. Vision therapy treated me with respect and empathy.

After a few minutes, I could feel the tense muscles around my eyes relaxing.

After the brief break, I tried again, doing exactly as instructed. Still double.

"Your eye tends to drift inward. Look away for a few seconds and then try again. Try to see peripherally while looking straight ahead."

"This is impossible."

I suddenly felt a weird sensation in my head as the image unexpectedly came into focus.

"It's single now, but it feels strange."

"Your brain is making new connections!" Evelyn excitedly said. "Great work. Now take a minute, then let's try a different picture."

CHICKEN THERAPY

No rest for the weary indeed.

I left that session exhausted but pleased with my progress. It felt so good to accomplish something through hard work, especially on a computer screen.

***

A few weeks after the hearing, Carl called to say that he had received the official notice from Social Security that the appeal was successful and that my Social Security Disability claim had been accepted. I would start receiving monthly checks in a few weeks, along with two-thirds of the back Social Security lump sum owed to me since I had stopped working. It felt as though a huge weight had been lifted. Now I could continue with my therapy and regain more control over my life.

When I told Jon the good news, he was as excited as I was.

"Finally, a break. All your hard work is paying off."

He was right. The judgment was bittersweet. It meant we'd get financial relief. It also meant I probably would not be able to get back to my career.

***

Nine months after my first vision therapy session, it was time for another evaluation.

"Congratulations!" Dr. Roser said after doing the usual set of tests. "I'm happy to report that your symptoms have stabilized. Your brain's ability to put together the images of both eyes has improved to the point that you don't need any more therapy. After one more session where we will teach you some additional maintenance exercises to strengthen your ability to manage the effects of the injury in the future, you'll be done."

"That's great news…I think."

"It is. Your progress has been amazing."

CHICKEN THERAPY

"What if I continued the therapy? I seem to have so much more to do. Would that make a difference?"

"Not significantly enough to justify the cost. Think about how much your quality of life has gotten better compared to nine months ago."

I had to admit that my symptoms and life had drastically improved as a result of the vision therapy.

"You're right. I guess I was expecting that if I continued the sessions, I'd get cured eventually."

"That's a common reaction. Some people with less severe injuries often feel that way. In your case, vision therapy has given you the skills to cope with the condition and thrive. It's the great benefit of this therapy. I wish more people knew about it."

"Thank you for all you've done." We shook hands.

After my last session, Evelyn said, "It was a pleasure working with you, Chris. Keep up the exercises and stay in touch. All the best. Spread the word about VT to anyone you think might benefit."

"I will. I appreciate all your help." We hugged.

On the drive home, I couldn't stop thinking about what she'd said about spreading the word. More people needed to know about vision therapy, including doctors and therapists. Maybe I could help by sharing my experience with others and getting the word out about this amazing therapy.

As I sit amongst the fruit trees,

and ponder and observe,

It finally dawns upon me,

Exactly what had just occurred.

CHAPTER 24

I slowly adjusted to my new lifestyle. Now that the regular sessions of vision therapy were over, I made a point of keeping up with my exercises. When I got distracted and forgot to do them or overdid my activities, my vision regressed. It would always be a harsh reminder that although I had learned to manage my symptoms, the underlying problem would always be lingering in the background. I had to remain vigilant.

I no longer woke up every day feeling depressed and helpless with no purpose or hope. Now that I was feeling able to engage in more activities outside my home, I got back into leading a life governed by an actual schedule, as I once had. I had always enjoyed keeping fit and swimming, so I decided to join the local rec center's water aerobics class.

The indoor pool was beautiful, and the rest of the facility was inviting. The weekly classes added to my exercise regimen, and I even started swimming a bit. Our group of women was warm and friendly and helped me to reconnect socially.

I slowly went back to holding regular large family gatherings as well, being careful to give myself plenty of time to prepare. I made sure that the following day's schedule was free to allow myself the opportunity to relax, do my exercises, and generally recover.

My parents, both past eighty, were healthy but slowly declining. I made sure to spend plenty of time with them. Jade and Adrianna now both lived locally, and since I could drive more easily, we saw each of them more often.

Balancing these activities with intermittent rest brought me back to a semblance of my normal life before the accident. I continued to write in my journal, recounting the new lease on life vision therapy had given me. I did miss teaching. As I grew more confident, I remained hopeful that I'd get back to it someday.

Successfully managing my new way of living required perseverance and discipline. I made a point of setting a time when I paid bills or used my computer. Spending time with my now flock always gave me the outlet I needed to rest my eyes and brain on the days I overdid things, and there were many.

******

The next major issue was the accident lawsuit. Two and a half years later, it was still "in process." It had been months since I had informed Henry that my social security case had been settled. He said he still hadn't heard back from the insurance company concerning the deposition or the hearing date. I got the sense that if I didn't stay in touch with him regularly, there'd be little progress.

Finally, he called to say that the date for the deposition by the defense attorneys had been set, and he had received the list of four doctors I had to see in the coming weeks to assess my condition: psychologist (again), neuro-psychologist, neuro-ophthalmologist, and orthopedist before the depositions.

Henry warned me to stay off social media as the defense would be watching and waiting for any evidence that would nullify my claims, such as posts about a new job, vacation photos, or other activities that would make me appear unaffected by the accident. I rarely posted on social media, so I was not worried about it. I had heard stories about insurance companies hiring private investigators to follow people around to see if they were faking their injuries, and that made me a bit paranoid. It was a stressful time. I frequently felt as though I was the one on trial, not the victim of the accident.

For the next few weeks, I concentrated on surviving the numerous doctor visits mandated by the defense. Each visit with a doctor was at least an hour away. It almost seemed as if the insurance company made it as difficult as possible.

The visits were perfunctory. Each doctor had me fill out a form describing my injuries, then did a short exam and signed off. I expected them to be much tougher, looking for ways to deny my complaint. It was all part of the system. However, the last visit with the neuro-ophthalmologist was particularly taxing.

He put me through the same grueling tests on the computer I had experienced years ago, which forced my symptoms to return so badly that I couldn't finish it. It was demeaning to have to prove that my condition was serious and permanent. It took me days afterward to recover with exercises and rest.

"I'm done with the visits," I told Henry after the last visit.

"Good. The ball can get rolling now."

"What happens next?"

"Now that the doctors have done their reports, we will begin with the next phase of what is called the discovery phase, the deposition. It will be held in a conference room here at my office."

"Their lawyers will do the questioning. You will be asked to verify facts regarding the accident, your injuries, and your inability to work. They will be looking for anything that contradicts any information we have given them. They'll try to trip you up. I'll be there to make sure they don't get out of line. Your husband may be questioned as well."

"Is there anything that we should or shouldn't say? Do we need to do anything to prepare?" I wanted to avoid the experience I had with Carl and Social Security.

"No. Just answer the question as briefly as possible. Be honest. Be confident and clear. Be yourselves. It should go well."

I hoped he was right.

On the day of the deposition, I awoke with a start when my alarm went off at 5:00 a.m. I immediately jumped out of bed and headed for the shower. My vision was good, and I was feeling positive, if a bit nervous.

As Jon watched me zoom around the kitchen, putting away dishes and barking orders at him to check on the coop before we left, he realized that for the first time in over two years, a glimpse of the old me was showing.

"You seem psyched for this thing," he said.

"I guess I am."

We watched a few YouTube videos on how to prepare for a deposition and reviewed all my medical records. I wanted to feel as confident as possible during the deposition.

Jon said that if they questioned him, he would make sure that they understood the horror I'd been through the past two years. I loved him for always having my back but was a bit worried that he might get carried away. Maybe that would be a good thing. I had no idea.

I had carefully planned my outfit: black dress pants, a light blue blouse, and a matching light blue blazer. Tan pumps and minimal jewelry created the look I was after: confident and professional.

Jon was handsome in a suit and tie. He normally wore work clothes, and his appearance caught my eye.

"You clean up pretty well," I said, teasing as we were about to leave.

"Gotta keep up with my pretty wife."

I remembered why I had fallen in love with him. We were so good together, always had been.

After a good breakfast, we walked to the car, past the coop. Jon had fed the birds and shooed them inside earlier, as we'd be gone the whole day. Before entering the car, I took a deep breath and looked around. As I inhaled the fresh air and took in the beauty of the day and my surroundings, it felt good.

CHICKEN THERAPY

The traffic was bad, and finding a parking place was almost impossible. Even though we had allotted two hours for what was usually an hour-long trip to Henry's Philadelphia office, we were almost late. We finally found a space and hurriedly walked toward the office building.

"How are you feeling?" Jon asked, holding my hand.

"Ready." It was the first time we'd been there. Thank God there was no revolving door.

"May I help you?" a man at the front desk asked.

"We're here for a deposition," I said. "Henry Arsdale is our attorney. Chris and Jon Helm."

He looked at his screen. "Yes, his office is on twelve. The elevator is on your right."

My good side, I thought.

I was a bit surprised when we entered Henry's office. It was small and a bit shabby. His secretary sat at an old desk to the left of the inner door.

"You must be the Helms," she said. "Go right in. Henry is waiting for you."

"Good morning," Henry said. "Good to see you after all this time. How was the drive?"

"Pretty bad," Jon said. "We just made it."

"Yeah, it's always congested at this time of day, but no worries. The insurance team hasn't arrived yet."

Henry was dressed sharply in a nice suit. His desk was cluttered with stacks of folders and papers that he shuffled through until he found ours.

"Let's talk for a few minutes before the attorneys get here," he said, leading us to the small conference room where the deposition would take place. We sat at a long, oblong table. Moving between rooms in the unfamiliar surroundings made my double vision kick in a bit. I had to close my eyes to help get it under control.

CHICKEN THERAPY

"Chris, are you okay?" Jon asked.

I nodded. "Just had to rest my eyes for a second. Any chance I could get a cup of coffee?"

"Make that two," Jon added. "Sure."

He called out to his secretary to bring them up.

Henry coached us on a wide variety of questions, most about my job, the various treatments I had received, including vision therapy, my shoulder injury, and the effect the accident had on our lives and finances. I felt prepared having gone through a similar process with the Social Security judge. Jon would need to wait in Henry's office until it was his turn. I was a bit worried about Jon. I could see that he bristled at some of the questions. I hoped he could remain calm.

"Remember, answer the question asked as briefly as possible. Don't ramble on or share any extraneous details."

After the prep session and the coffee, I was feeling better. We sat in the conference room while Henry arranged the papers. A stenographer joined us at a small table to the side of the conference table.

A short time later, Henry's secretary ushered the defense attorney into the room.

I took a deep breath. *Be confident, you got this.*

The lawyer was young, wore an expensive suit, and seemed a bit nervous.

"Sorry, I'm a bit late. The traffic was terrible."

"No problem," Henry said and stood. "Henry Arsdale, the attorney representing Mrs. Christine Helm."

"Steve Nessim, attorney for the defense. Let's get started."

Mr. Nessim took a seat opposite us. He signaled to the stenographer to begin taking the notes. He restated his name and the name of his client, the insurance company, and the purpose of the deposition. Henry stated his name, his role, and my name. Then Mr. Nessim went down the list of procedural rules.

CHICKEN THERAPY

"Excuse me. Could you repeat that last one?" I asked.

"Please don't interrupt the procedure, Mrs. Helm," he responded.

"My client is just trying to make sure she fully understands the process," Henry said in my defense.

"We've got a tight schedule, Mr. Arsdale. We need to stick to the procedure."

"Understood. Please repeat the last procedural step for Mrs. Helm, then we can get on with it."

Angry, Mr. Nessim did so, then began the questioning.

I settled in and answered each question concisely. I felt good about my responses. After I was done, an hour or so later, I was asked to wait outside while Jon's deposition took place. The door was partially open, and I could hear bits and pieces of muffled conversation.

As I listened, I could tell Jon's answers were not as short and to the point as mine had been. After a few minutes, I thought I could hear Jon's tone change. He was losing his composure, getting loud and agitated. Henry had to intervene a few times to keep him on track.

After the deposition was over, the defense lawyer left the office without the courtesy of a goodbye. We sat with Henry to get a sense of how it went.

"I'd say it went fairly well. We got a little off-topic at times, but all in all, we got all the major points across."

"Will you get to question the driver?"

"Afraid not. Her role is well-documented. It's all about your claim with the insurance company at this point. If we go to trial, she may take the stand. It's unlikely. We'll have to see."

"What do you mean 'if' we go to trial? I thought that was the next step?" Jon said.

"Now that they have all the information and know we are serious about pursuing the claim, they may decide to offer to settle to avoid a trial. If I hear anything, I'll let you know."

CHICKEN THERAPY

"Thanks," I said.

Jon and I made our way back to the car.

"I'm glad that's over," he said. "That lawyer had some attitude."

"He's young, and I thought he was just doing his job." "I guess you're right."

"All we can do is wait to see what's next and get back to our lives."

Life is not a game of give and take,

The prize not up for grabs.

Life is just about survival,

Getting by and bouncing back.

CHAPTER 25

One afternoon, several weeks later, I returned to the garden to do some weeding. Hearing a squawk, I turned my attention to the hill. Lady Gaga had determined that a butterfly was a direct threat to her and couldn't decide if she should flee to the coop or stay hidden in the weeds. I laughed when she jumped straight up, flapped her wings, and sprinted for the cover of a nearby bush.

She then hid her head in the bush and stood frozen like a statue, as if by hiding from the problem, it would just go away. She hadn't realized that by flapping her wings, she had scared the butterfly away and inadvertently solved her problem. I wondered if she would learn that she had the power to scare away any further butterflies.

Lady Gaga's experience gave me an idea.

Dr. Roser and Evelyn's parting comments to me about how little people knew about the benefits of vision therapy never left my mind. That therapy saved my sanity when traditional medical practice had not, yet most people and doctors still knew little about it. While there was already a great deal of information about VT on the internet, most of it was technical and difficult to understand. Even most doctors didn't think to explore it as an option for their patients. Millions of people suffering from concussion injuries and other challenges didn't know it existed. They needed to know that there is something that could help them take control of their problem.

At that moment, I had an insight. It was the kind of feeling you know deep down is right but have no idea why; the kind of idea that seemed so obvious you wondered why you never thought about it before. Maybe there was something I could do to spread the word about vision therapy after all, to help people flap their wings to help them with their issues.

CHICKEN THERAPY

I walked briskly back to the house, ran up the steps to the bedroom, and rummaged through the closet to find the large black cardboard box where I kept all my crayon journals and many of the documents from doctors I'd saved since the accident.

If I could organize all this information, I could share my story with others in a book and help them navigate the crazy world of vision challenges I knew all too well. Most importantly, I wanted to herald the benefits of vision therapy in a way people could easily understand. Vision therapy had given me back my life and I had to share my story.

I quickly realized that the task of organizing all those random documents and journal entries was enormous. I knew I had to find a way. I took the box into the study and began the work.

It soon became clear that I needed a larger space to work. The desk in the study was too small. I needed space to spread out the large pads and other materials and begin work on the book itself.

Each day I spent with all the materials, I realized there were too many distractions in the house. Every time I tried to focus, I got a phone call, the dog would need attention, or some chore would give me an excuse to stop.

Jon could see the problem. When he came home, he found me surrounded by piles of paper. "You need a place to go, whenever you want, outside of the house, to work on this idea."

"I guess I do. Too bad the barn is in such bad shape."

"It's too big anyway."

"I need my own coop."

"I have an idea. We could buy one of those big, prefab storage sheds and set it up as your office, outside. I'd insulate it, get a heater, a desk, your nephew can wire it for power and…"

Jon was off to the races with the idea. It would be exactly what I needed: my own she-shed shack for my project.

"Where do you want it?"

CHICKEN THERAPY

We walked outside. I glanced up on the hill at the adorable wooden coop with the attached run Jon had built. It was about fifty yards from the barn.

"How about in that space between the barn and the coop?"

"That will work. I can put windows on the side so you can view the chickens and then more windows in the front so you can see the yard."

"Perfect!" I exclaimed.

A week later, a shed was delivered and put in place. The following week, Jon installed some windows he found on Craigslist. My nephew, Jason, connected the electricity. It was all coming together.

"Come inside the shed with me," Jon said.

"Why?"

"We need to decide where to place a desk and shelves."

"And I'll need an easel to put the pads on to write."

"I can do that."

I found a large throw rug and desk chair at a local thrift store. Two weeks later, it was ready.

"It's perfect," I said. "Thanks so much." I gave Jon a big kiss.

The girls helped me move and organize all my materials into what I now called "my writing shack." Then I began the arduous task of pulling all the bits and pieces, random thoughts, and information together into one coherent narrative.

Through trial and error, I learned to schedule the time I spent writing on days with no outside appointments. I found my limit for writing was only a few hours at a time, provided I spread them out using the 20-20-20 rule. I sometimes got lost in my writing and forgot to set the timer. My aching eye muscles and double vision reminded me to take breaks. It was frustrating because I grew to love the process and hated having to stop.

My method of using large artist pads and crayons continued to be the easiest, least stressful way for me to put down my thoughts.

CHICKEN THERAPY

Jon had set up a sturdy easel stand for me to use. Referring to my old journals, I would fill up a sheet, then just flip it over and start a fresh one. Once I had accumulated several pages, I'd attempt to transcribe them onto my laptop. That was the hardest part, as I had to limit my computer time.

I found an app that had an improved talk-to-text feature and used it frequently. One day, I knew that I needed to read some of the materials I transcribed and knew that my eyes would not cooperate. I hated not being able to read everything I had just created in one sitting. I knew that writing was all about re-writing and editing.

That night at dinner, I shared my frustrations with Jon.

"I wish someone could read and record what I had transcribed, and then I could listen to it and make changes, instead of reading the entire thing."

"Maybe there's an app for that."

"What?"

"You are the technology whiz. Maybe there's an app for that."

"Why didn't I think of that?"

The next day, I found an app that allowed you to download documents and then it would read it back. I could follow along and edit in segments. It was fifty dollars a month. I shared the discovery with Jon.

"I knew you'd find a way. Buy it, we can find a way to cut a few corners."

"Thank you," I said with tears in my eyes.

"What's wrong?"

"I am just so happy! I'm finally doing something that could make a difference instead of just surviving. I missed that feeling. That's why I got into teaching."

On writing days, I fill my backpack with my laptop and snacks and head up to my shack. Before entering, I stop by the coop, open

CHICKEN THERAPY

its door, and watch my flock excitedly run down the ramp. They then crowd around the gate, waiting for me to open it, pecking and squawking as they frantically push their way to freedom.

As I walk to the shack just beyond, they follow me, expecting snacks. I shoo them away as I open the door to my little world and close it. I can hear them softly clucking outside for a few minutes until they realize I'm not coming out, so they leave to free range. The happy, quiet atmosphere of my shack, surrounded by the familiarity of my chickens, provides the environment I need to continue my writing.

Writing gave me an entirely new perspective. In finding my voice to record my story, I could finally see the proverbial forest for the trees. I could see a clear path through my experiences to my eventual recovery through vision therapy.

I finally figured out that life isn't about being a victim of what had happened to me or the fairness of the system. It is about digging deep, persevering, and fighting back. It is about learning to slow down and observe all the wisdom the world has to offer. It is about accepting, not avoiding, fear and pain and finding a way to get through it.

If you really want to know,

How the world works, what makes it spin,

Observe nature at its finest,

Then follow that voice from within.

CHAPTER 26

About a month after the depositions, Henry called. "A hearing date has been set at the federal courthouse in Allentown."

"I guess they didn't decide to settle."

"The purpose of the hearing is to try to settle the case with help from a judge and avoid going to a full jury trial."

"What should we expect?"

"You've approved the information from our economist about the amount we're looking for. I will present it at the hearing. Most likely, they will counter with another figure. Your role is to accept or reject their offer. If we reject it, then we continue to negotiate. If we can't agree, then the judge will call for a jury trial. The trial would most likely be in about six months. However, it rarely gets to that point in my experience. No one wants the time and expense of trial. You may want to think about what is the lowest offer that you are willing to accept."

I discussed it with Jon. He felt strongly that the original figure from Henry's economist was justified.

"What if they don't agree? It's a huge amount. Maybe we should figure out what might be a compromise we could accept before the hearing as Henry suggested?"

"No point second guessing ourselves. We need to go through the process to see what they come up with. It could be something we could live with."

Practical as always, Jon's advice gave us a solid approach. I tried to remain hopeful.

***

On a brisk November day, Jon and I approached our destination, the hearing, after a ten-minute uphill walk from the parking garage.

CHICKEN THERAPY

The federal building was daunting. The architecture gave it an air of historic authority and grandeur. I told myself to be composed and confident as we were guided through the resplendent building to the courtroom.

Henry was waiting for us. I prayed that because Jon and I had always tried to live a life where our choices were made using good morals and values, I prayed that justice would prevail, and we would get a fair settlement.

After introductions, the judge explained the series of events that would take place. The head lawyer for the insurance company, Richard Foster, was accompanied by Steve Nessim and a third colleague. That's a lot of lawyers, I thought nervously.

"I will preside over the settlement process until there is a resolution. Failing that, I will set a date for a jury trial," the judge concluded.

When the short introduction ended, Jon and I were ushered by Henry into a stuffy windowless room, decorated in cheap brown paneling and tattered furniture.

"You and Jon will now wait here, while I meet with the defense team and judge to present our demand and hear their counteroffer. I will then come back to you to hear what you think."

An hour later, Henry returned to our room with the first settlement offer from the insurance company.

"You are joking," Jon said. "That won't even pay our current bills, let alone compensate us for the lost income and the ordeal Chris has gone through."

"It's only the first offer. I'm obligated to present it to you. They always start very low. We need to remain firm with the amount we worked out. It's all part of the process."

This process went on for hours with some progress made. Although their second offer was nowhere near our amount, it was closer.

CHICKEN THERAPY

Henry walked in and announced that we were given a brief recess for lunch.

"This may take some time," Henry said. "They are pretty firm. You may want to get some lunch. There's a place across the street."

"Will you join us?" I asked.

"Love to, but I stay around here."

On our way back from lunch, I heard laughing and looked through the open door of what appeared to be a break room. The judge, our lawyer, and the defense team lawyers were sitting around having lunch and chatting like old friends.

"What's with that?" I said. "Aren't they all supposed to be adversaries?"

Jon shrugged. "I guess they're here so often that they know each other well. It shouldn't affect the outcome."

"I hope you're right."

Once back in the little waiting room, exhausted, my mind began to wander. Why did it seem that I was no longer a victim of a wrongdoer, deserving of compensation? I had become a pawn in a strange game of chess.

I realized that, unlike chess players, these opponents were not against each other, they were working together towards a mutually beneficial outcome. Unaware of our role in the game, Jon and I had become isolated. We were on our own in this world governed by money and power, yet still carefully hidden behind the facade of truth and justice that created it.

The process took all afternoon. Henry would repeatedly come back and report each change in the settlement. As the hours passed, the amount they offered slowly crept higher. It never approached our original figure.

After what seemed to be a particularly long negotiating session, Henry finally walked back in.

"I don't think they will budge. They stipulated that this was their final offer. You can either accept it or we can go to trial."

"How long will that take?" Jon asked.

"Depends on the judge's schedule. It could take six months to get a court date. Then another few months to pick the jury and get started."

"That's almost another year," I said.

"Well, despite time, going to a jury trial is risky. Your case is unusual. It's not like you lost a leg or something that tangible. Most people haven't heard of your kind of injury or wouldn't understand how serious it is. And, as you seem to be coping with it effectively, they might think it is not worth as large an award as you are asking for. You could even get nothing. It's up to you."

"What you're telling us is that after all we've gone through, there's a chance we would wind up with no compensation for Chris's pain and suffering, not to mention our financial losses?"

"I've seen it happen. It's always a risk. It's my job to lay out all the options. It's up to you to instruct me how to proceed."

"Could you give us a few minutes to discuss this?" I asked.

"Sure. I'll be back in about ten minutes or so." He left.

"After all this," Jon said, "we were the ones who had to compromise. It's not fair. Maybe he just wants to get it over with to get his commission."

"Maybe, but he's gone through all this before. What if he's right? What if we reject this, go to trial, and get a jury who does not understand the impact of my injuries? It is possible that we could get nothing."

"It's your decision. You're the one who has suffered more than anyone."

"I need this to end. I don't want to go through another year of waiting, followed by a grueling jury trial. I need to make a fresh start, with whatever amount of money we have."

He took my hand. "Okay, let's do it."

When Henry returned, we told him our decision. "I think you made the right choice, given the circumstances."

He left to inform the bailiff that we were ready to meet with the judge. We were escorted back to the courtroom, where the judge, all of the lawyers, and a few other court officials were milling around preparing for the outcome. The defense team was positioned at a table on the left, and we were instructed to sit at one on the right. The judge was seated behind an impressive wooden bench at the front of the large room.

"What is your decision?" he asked.

Henry rose. "My clients have agreed to accept the settlement offer, Your Honor."

"So noted." He read the settlement statement and handed the document to us to sign, then to the defense to inspect and sign as well. Next, we each received a copy of the signed documents. Lastly, the judge adjourned the proceeding and left.

As we were preparing to leave, Foster, the head defense lawyer, walked over to greet me. "I am very sorry about your accident and what you've gone through. Good luck to you," he said sincerely, extending his hand.

I didn't know what to say. He and his company had been the enemy for so long. It seemed weird to shake hands and forget about it all.

"Thank you," I said softly as we shook hands. I didn't know what to feel. Was this finally over?

Henry followed us out. "I'll be in touch when we get the final check. Thanks for your patience with this whole process."

We thanked him and went home.

Early that January, I received a phone call from a colleague at my former school. She had recently accepted a new job as a math teacher at a local public school just when COVID hit. I knew the

CHICKEN THERAPY

school. It wasn't that far away. It was larger than my old school and had many of the same courses.

"The school was trying to institute a new online teaching system for remote learning. Many of the teachers were having trouble adapting. We desperately need someone who could help. I thought of you and how great you were with technology at our old school. When I mentioned you to the principal, he told me to contact you."

Her words made me feel good.

"Thanks for thinking of me. I'm not sure I'm interested in going back to full-time work."

"The system isn't all that different from the one at our school. You'd be more of a consultant, not a full-time person—just until the system was up and running and everyone was trained."

I began to get a little excited. *It sounded like my old job, only less demanding. I was feeling pretty good. My symptoms were minimal. Maybe I can do this!*

"Sounds challenging. Let me think about it."

"Great. Thanks. I'll let the principal know you're interested. It would be fun working with you again." She gave me the link to the online application.

When Jon got home from work that night, I told him about the potential job.

"You're doing so well; maybe you should go for it. It's only temporary and not far from home."

His confidence inspired me to pursue it.

The next morning, I sat at my laptop and clicked on the link for the application. It required me to dig up references, addresses, and details about my other teaching jobs. I had to find my teaching certificate, arrange background checks, and write an essay. It meant a lot of work on the computer, so I had to pace myself. Even with the 20-20-20 rule, it took all day.

"How'd the application go?" Jon asked.

"It was complicated. I'm still not finished."

"You look tired."

"Yes, I am. My eyes hurt."

"You rest. I'll make dinner," he said.

The next morning, my symptoms were slightly better but still present. I tried to do a few exercises and relax. Although that helped a little, I still wasn't feeling up to resuming the computer work on the application.

"There is no way I can go back to the computer today. I did way too much yesterday."

Jon put down his coffee cup. "I know you want to do this. It's a great opportunity for you. But…"

I knew what he was going to say.

"Well, don't get mad. If you had this kind of reaction after working at home for hours on the computer, it might be tough to take on this tech job at the school."

"You may be right. If I pace myself and do my exercises, maybe it could work. We could use the extra money."

"It's up to you, but I think you should consider how it would affect your health. It's a lot of pressure with everyone scrambling because of the pandemic."

Even though I knew he was right, the prospect of going back to work was so attractive to me. "I'm going to see if I can finish the application and then see how I feel."

"Okay. I'm with you no matter what you decide."

I did a few more exercises, took care of the coop, and then tried to resume my work on the application. After a short time, my symptoms started again.

That clinched it. I had to recognize my limits. Sadly, I called my friend to tell her that I had decided not to apply for the job.

"Too bad. I know you'd do a terrific job."

CHICKEN THERAPY

"Thanks. I appreciate the opportunity." We made a date to have lunch soon.

It took a few days for me to shake the sorrow from the reality that had sunk in. Even though I had gotten a good handle on how to manage my symptoms, I now had to recognize that my condition was permanent, and getting back to work full-time was not in the cards.

My decision to not return to outside work turned out to be a godsend. Jon had been considering starting his own consulting business. He had a great reputation and had been building contacts for years. He felt he could make more money on his own rather than working at his present company. There was some money left over from the insurance settlement to start the business.

We developed a plan. Jon started building a customer base in the evenings and on the weekends. I did the back-office work of securing a business ID number and setting up some systems for billing, bookkeeping, marketing, and creating a website. I worked on the plan no more than an hour or two a day, making sure that I took a break every twenty minutes.

It all started to come together. When we had a critical mass of projects, Jon gave notice, and the new business was born.

Things were tight for a few months before the business generated a steady income. Jon took the phone calls and did estimates for the customers. I worked a few hours a day, a few days a week on the accounts and fielding queries on the website. We worked well as a team, and the business prospered.

It felt great being able to make an equal contribution, on my terms. It also allowed me the time to continue the work on my book.

One evening, my eyes tired and head aching, I went out to close up the coop for the night. I felt a twinge of anger at myself for once again overextending myself that day. The coop had remained my steadfast refuge.

CHICKEN THERAPY

After doing a head count, I turned over a bucket and sat on it to watch the birds enjoy their last few moments of freedom. Jack, Sally, and Sandy were contentedly wandering the run, while Brie and Gouda perched on a high branch Jon had installed for them. After a few minutes, I gently shooed the flock into the coop.

Orloff, now contentedly roosting beside Kevin, indicated her new status in the flock. She had held her ground against the bullies and had slowly, but passively, risen to the top. Ruby and Lady Gaga, on the other hand, rested far away from the others on the outcast roost. They had learned to find comfort in each other.

I looked at them all and smiled. Our flock had changed over the years—broody hens, chicks, rescues, and predators—all playing their part. Year after year, nature continued to deliver both good and bad circumstances, and the flock took it all in stride. They seemed to know that, no matter how hard they tried, they couldn't prevent bad things from happening.

The insights I gained from my flock gave me the courage to keep trying, despite all the challenges. They taught me that I didn't need to restore my old vision to find joy in life. I needed to find a new vision.

Most victims of a brain injury can't verbalize how they feel when the symptoms from their concussion or cranial nerve damage occur. Having no idea what is causing the symptoms or why they don't subside makes it difficult for them to explain their debilitating state. Vision therapy supplies the knowledge and tools to communicate and manage those symptoms effectively.

Maybe the darkness was here first, and the light came second. I still struggle to stay in the light, but evening always comes, and so does the night. But then comes another day and another light.

RESOURCES

To find a vision therapist near you:
Visit the Neuro-Optometric Rehabilitation Association at
https://nora.memberclicks.net/find-a-provider#/

To learn more about vision therapy, visit these sites:
The Neuro-Optometric Rehabilitation Association at
www.noravisionrehab.org.
The Optometric Extension Program Foundation at
www.oepf.org.
The College of Optometrists in Vision Development at
www.covd.org.

For financial assistance with vision therapy:
Contact an Office of Vocational Rehabilitation near you at
dli.pa.gov/Individuals/Disability-Services/ovr/Pages/default.aspx

www.ingramcontent.com/pod-product-compliance
Lightning Source LLC
Chambersburg PA
CBHW050526100526
44581CB00008B/142/J